THIS
MORTAL
COIL

THIS
MORTAL
COIL

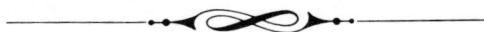

The Meaning
of Health and Disease

KENNETH L. VAUX

1817

Published in San Francisco by

HARPER & ROW, PUBLISHERS

New York, Hagerstown, San Francisco, London

FIRST EDITION

Designed by Jim Mennick

International Standard Book Number: 0–06–068856–4
Library of Congress Catalog Card Number: 77–7846

78 79 80 81 82 10 9 8 7 6 5 4 3 2 1

Contents

Foreword

Animals weakened by age or disease do not survive long
under natural conditions. They are likely to be abandoned by
their group and to die victims of environmental stresses or
predators. The ability to survive and to function in the wilder-
ness implies the possession of a high degree of biological fitness
to the total environment and of resistance to its dangers. This
state of adaptiveness is the basis of biological health; and significant departure from it results in some state of disease,
commonly followed by death within a short time. Biological
health implies, furthermore, that the organism under consideration is in a state compatible with its further anatomical and
physiological development and with the normal development
of its progeny. For example, the healthy female stores nu-
trients before the mating period and exhibits behavior patterns
exquisitely fitted to the care of the young. The attributes that
make for biological health therefore inevitably involve the future.

The mechanisms for adaptation to the present and to the
future are encoded in the genetic apparatus that defines each
species. Under natural conditions, these mechanisms are
adequate for the maintenance of health as long as the total
environment retains the essential characteristics that prevailed
during the evolutionary period when the species acquired its
distinctive characteristics. Biological health is a consequence of
evolutionary adaptation.

In the human species also, the states of health and disease correspond to the relative degrees of success or failure in the attempt to respond adaptively to environmental challenges. However, the relationships between human beings and their environment involve not only physicochemical forces but also—and chiefly—sociocultural factors that have little, if any, effect on the Darwinian mechanisms of evolution and that, consequently, do not generate biological instructions encoded in the genetic endowment. The study of Old Stone Age skeletons has revealed, for example, that certain Neanderthal people who had been severely crippled by accidents or by disease, and therefore were unable to fend for themselves, nevertheless did survive for several decades after suffering their handicaps. It can be surmised that, in some way, they had been supported by other members of their group instead of being abandoned, as they would have been in an animal society. In primitive as well as in advanced human societies, survival is therefore conditioned not only by the biological determinants of health and disease but also by sociocultural values.

Genetic instructions for adaptive responses to the environment naturally exist in the human species just as they do in other species, but they are rarely adequate for the usual conditions of human life. One of the characteristics of humankind is the urge to move into the unknown and to accept or even elect environmental conditions different from those which prevailed when *Homo sapiens* acquired its biological identity. The biological nature of the human species has not significantly changed since the Stone Age, but few are the human beings who live in a truly natural environment. Wherever human beings have settled, in fact, they have created conditions and ways of life different from those under which their biological evolution took place.

The changes in ways of life during prehistory and history make it clear that the state of adaptation to the toal environment inevitably changes with social evolution. For example, the biological aspects of adaptation to the hunter-gatherer life differed from those to agrarian societies, or to the first industrial revolution, or to the automation age. Social change, even when it means real progress, inevitably implies new dangers. Disease ensues whenever human beings fail, as they frequently do, to make rapidly enough the proper adaptive responses to the new environmental conditions they encounter in the course of their social explorations.

The prodigious diversity of requirements created by human occupations and aspirations makes it difficult to achieve the state of *mens sana in corpore sano* and even to formulate a definition of this health ideal. The kind of physical and mental health required by a young Jewish woman who has elected to live in an isolated kibbutz in Israel differs profoundly from that required by another Jewish woman of the same age and size who aspires to success as a fashion model in Paris or New York. Similarly, health does not mean the same thing for a European peasant operating a small family farm, a lumberjack in the Canadian Rockies, a New York City bus driver, a comedian expected to perform day after day in a crowded nightclub, or an ascetic monk worshiping God in the desert.

The criteria of health are thus vastly more complex in human life than they are in animal life because they involve not only biological determinants but also social values and individual choices that transcend biological necessity. For human beings, the nearest approach to health is a physical and mental state, fairly free of discomfort, that enables them to function as effectively and as long as possible in the pursuit of their social and cultural goals.

"Work is more important than life," Katherine Mansfield confided to the last pages of her journal. "By health, I mean the power to live a full, adult, living, breathing life in close contact with what I love—the earth and the wonders thereof. . . . *I*

want to be all that I am capable of becoming, so that I may be . . .
there's only one phrase that will do—*a child of the sun*." But the
sun is not merely a source of warmth, of light, of food, of
power. It is also the symbol of the aspirations through which
human beings consciously or unconsciously relate themselves
to the cosmic order.

Health could be described in purely biological terms if it
referred only to survival, physical vigor, and bodily comfort.
But an understanding of health requires also the theological
considerations discussed by Dr. Vaux, because few human beings are satisfied with biological health alone. Most people are
primarily concerned with purposive activities; they want to
develop some aspect of their humanity and to reach goals of
their choices. Such choices are made according to value systems that transcend biological criteria and that inevitably re-
flect philosophical attitudes concerning the meaning of human
life and its place in creation.

Preface

It is sophomoric and immodest to attempt to tackle again the question of the meaning of health and disease. The probing character of this book is justified only if my hunch is correct that the confusion over these issues constitutes a grave danger to our peace and sanity. The title of the book is a phrase from *Hamlet*. It indicates that what I am after are answers to perennial issues and that what I see developing is a medicine which merges the best of contemporary techniques with the best traditional understanding of our human frailty and need.

I have had the unique privilege of working in the unexcelled Texas Medical Center based in the Institute of Religion, whose history has been ever pioneering, and therefore precarious. To the trustees of the Institute, my colleagues Ron Sunderland and Art Travis, and especially to Julian Byrd, distinguished chaplain and most recently our director, I give my wholehearted thanks. Audrey Laymance and Wier Smith of the Institute have generously assisted the work in both form and content. Three physician colleagues—J. David Bybee, Glen Cunningham, and Jan VanEys—have helped immensely in pondering these questions, as have my colleagues in Ethics, Tris Engelhardt and Joseph Fletcher. Finally, to Walter Johnson, teacher and pastor, and to his family and friends, I say, thank you!

KENNETH L. VAUX

I
Introduction

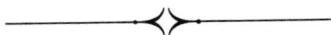

————◇————

Why God puts gallstones here, not there—
One man keeps his dinner down, another can't
These questions have used great minds down through the ages.
Job hollered to God and he got a promotion
and a nice write-up in the Bible.
Edith—I've been a good Christian all my life—ain't I?

—ARCHIE BUNKER, October 27, 1976

Why am I sick? Why do we suffer? Why do children die?
These universal and perennial questions of crisis are intimations of the more basic questions that we ask in wonder and in
pain.

When we ponder the enigmas of sickness and health, the
scientist and philosopher in each of us is especially concerned
with explanation: with smoothing out rough things. We will
not accept easy answers. Like Dostoevsky and Albert Camus,
our conscience is offended by easy and hasty theodicy. God
may have his ways; but we know we must not surrender but
probe, waiting for any glimmering of light to appear in this
dark night of evil. In fact, we deliberately defy both God and
Cosmos to present a meaningful order. In Robert Browning's
words, we "welcome each rebuff/ That turns earth's smooth-
ness rough . . ."; yet our dissatisfaction mounts as we continue
to reject the facile explanation in search of the deep.

Perhaps we should not be so bold as to reopen the theodicy
question.[1] How can we justify the ways of God to humanity?

The ancients were absorbed in pondering the meaning of suffering and physical evil; the Platonists, Epicureans, and Stoics
recommended responses of ecstasis, serenity, and self-control.
Theology could not disengage God from the problem. It gen-
erated the Iranean and Augustinian traditions, the former ac-
cepting pain as character building and the latter viewing pain
as fundamentally unreal. Classic writers like Dante and Milton
sought to explain divine justice in the face of natural and moral
evil. Modern writers not only despair of the answer but re-
pudiate the question. Yet the question persists; and in a culture
so obsessed with vitality and growth and so offended by degen-
eration and death, we are forced to construct a theodicy—or at
least an anthropolicy—in which we posit some rhyme and reason to the pain and joy of our existence. Even if the question of
the purpose of God has receded from modern life, the ways of
human beings need to be justified.

What has been the shape of our trust in God as it bears on the
experience of sickness? Traditionally, we have seen God as a
protector and healer. God's blessing conveys immunization
and salvation. He preserves our life (Genesis 45). Neither sun,
nor moon, nor pestilence shall smite us (Psalm 121). The Lord
is shield and defender (Psalm 35). He heals our disease (Isaiah
53). The theodicy question in its deeper dimension concerns
the sense of having been abandoned that we feel when we are
not protected, when we do not get well. To succumb to profound illness and death is to lose freedom, to experience bond-
age, to feel forsaken. The experience of health and disease
thus forces the reconstruction and clarification of theology.
Conversely, the basic understandings of God, humanity, and
the world that we hold tend to color the ways we interpret these
experiences.

Being children of the late twentieth century, we are cast into
great confusion as we search out these questions. We have
inherited a tradition of belief and value which is profoundly

challenged by new knowledge. The knowledge of how and why things happen has often stripped us of such comfortable rationalizations as "It is God's will," "that's mother nature," "His number was up!" We now stand numb before the enigma of sickness and pain; and while the position may be morally mature, it is frightening to find absurdity at the depths.

The new bewildering innocence has emotive and rational dimensions. We are offended by the hasty attribution of pain to the divine will. In a moving scene in the splendid television series, "The Adams Chronicles," Abigail and John are riding home in the carriage following the burial of their infant son. The boy had died during the cold winter, and John tries to comfort his wife by recalling the words of her pastor father at the funeral. "Remember your father's words, Abby. God has his purpose." "He may," says Abigail, "but I hope I never find it out!" Any modern theodicy must embrace our critical awareness that "this need not have been," along with the deeper peace the sense of providence bestows.

At the cultural level, the rational tension is found where traditional belief meets the sciences of nature and of human life. Charles Raven, the British naturalist-theologian, has devoted much thought to this problem and interprets it in this way:

> The cause of our bewilderment . . . is that mankind has for three hundred years at least been losing its compass-bearings, has been finding itself increasingly confounded with an underlying conflict between the traditional, ancient, venerable and impressive religions of the world and the new outlook on the universe and upon mankind and upon man's most intimate and searching experiences which the development of the modern scientific structure has inevitably produced.[2]

This book is motivated by the conviction that the crisis, which is both personal and cultural, is beginning to precipitate its resolution in new insights. The natural, scientific, and theological quests for the truth about human beings and the meaning of their experience are converging. It is where the life sciences and medicine converge with theology that we may experience the most significant breakthroughs in human knowledge in the years ahead. The following discussion of a theology of health and disease seeks to convey the insights emerging in that convergence.

This book is a sequel to my earlier work *Biomedical Ethics*.[3] It might also have been a preface. The questions about the evaluation of biomedical interventions have forced us to consider the fundamentals of ethics. The questions of what to do in crisis situations throw us back to the themes of the origin, nature, and destiny of human life. Although the intellectual crisis of the modern world has made metaphysical and theological reflection more problematic, the character and urgency of the real questions we face necessitate the inquiry.

One characteristic of the intellectual crisis we are now experiencing is that our simplistic schemes of explanation are yielding to richer concepts, more reflective of the real nature of things. In the explanation of disease, for example, we have labored for most of a century under the mistaken idea, born in the spirit of scientific positivism, that causation and description of everything could be framed in mechanistic, materialistic language, and that the process of progressive scientific illumination would gradually dispel the necessity for all dimensions of transcendence and spirit as explanatory factors.

Most of the philosophic misadventures that introduce scientific textbooks, most histories of medicine that venture normative judgments, uncritically expound such scientistic naiveté. Walther Riese begins his otherwise superb study, *The Conception of Disease*, with the statement: "The road from primitive to rational thought has to be sought and rediscovered anew by each generation . . . nor is any generation . . . protected against the danger of relapsing into early concepts, once the final stage is reached."[4]

The thrill of working in a great medical center where health and disease are not only thought about but experienced is that we know we have not reached any final stage. We are groping toward understanding. We can begin at long last to synthesize the insights of biomedicine, psychology, and theology on these questions. We can see both the wisdom of traditions and the limitation of the new science. We can begin to see that the older Comtian interpretation—that we have moved from superstitious through theistic to scientific explanations of nature and human life—has been convincingly questioned.

Progressive enlightenment, so imbedded in the current biomedical philosophy, sees the late medieval outlook and the New England puritan ethos, indeed any cultural vestige of a spirited or purposive world view, as a dark age seething with demonology and witchcraft. This progressive approach never considers the critical subtleties of those periods expressed in the genius of Albertus Magnus, Cusanus, Bacon, Mendel, the Mathers, Edwards, or Teilhard—all leaders of the church and scientific pioneers. In order to tear away from the age of faith, the age of reason and enlightenment developed what Jung has called a "murderous intellect." Fortunately, the dogmatism and mental vengeance of this position, often as constricting as those of the inquisition, are now waning and a new mood of unbiased inquiry is beginning. Modern science and medicine were born in the spirit of the Renaissance, when an anthropology of freedom and possibility contrasted vividly with ecclesiastical anthropologies. The latter, by accenting the human tragedy, set in motion decades of censorship, persecution, and distrust of the finer capacities of the human spirit. We can understand why science took the antireligious and anticlerical stance which endures to the present day. But we can also now see the need to move beyond this attitude. We can see the essential wisdom in both science and religion. We can envisage an age of creativity wherein a noble enterprise can be fashioned on a fundamental understanding of human beings which is at once pioneering and yet realistic about their limitations.

We are now free to explore the wide-ranging and complex understandings of the nature of health and disease that the phenomena merit. We can incorporate with new satisfaction the theological (spiritual and moral) and psychological dimensions, indeed the total ecological meaning, of health and disease.

In this book the contours of a modern theology of health and disease are outlined. Three steps are followed in the analysis. First, the traditional understanding of the meaning of health and disease is described. I contend that a constellation of meanings can be discerned, common to primitive and contemporary folk medicine, Judaic and Hippocratic views of health, and the traditional understanding of our culture up to the nineteenth century. This Tradition is repudiated and abandoned in the modern era, and an Experiment is begun. The second section of the book characterizes the Experiment, a period and mood which is just now coming to its conclusion, transmuting to a renovated constellation of meanings which blend Tradition and Experiment.

The scientific revolution had to take place to release our understanding of health and disease from fallacious meanings with which the Tradition had encrusted it. But the Experiment itself has gone down some blind alleys. The thrill of the present intellectual upheaval is that we are casting off what one writer has called "the constrictions of a mechanistic legacy."[5]

The final part of the book searches out the glimmerings on the horizon that suggest where we are going. These beacons of the future, I contend, are leading us to recapture the valid elements of the Tradition, integrating them with a new conceptualization of health and disease in their natural and transcending significance. What will emerge will be not the Tradition warmed over, nor a return to censorship and witch-hunting, though those dangers are always possible. What will emerge is a Renovation, a new structure of meaning that we will recognize as being perennially true. It will first emerge as common sense to individuals. It will then begin to reshape the structures of health care in our society. As I tried to suggest in *Biomedical Ethics*, a sense of the normative power of the past, together with an acute ethical perception of the present imperative, can best serve us as we approach the profound choices of our future.

What prompts me to structure the argument in this way? René Dubos has argued forcefully that we need not abandon our Judeo-Christian world view in order to come to grips with the modern scientific world view and give moral guidance to the uses we make of the derivative technologies. The environmental crisis, he claims, will not be resolved by abandoning Christianity and fleeing to the gurus of eastern nature mysticism.

With Helmut Thielicke I would go further to claim that a Judeo-Christian concept of nature has given rise to western history and to the scientific world view. Dubos finds in the Benedictines a mature world view and positive valuation of the place of human beings in the world. This religious tradition has also formed our moral awareness. This civilization cannot survive, let alone flourish, without the sustaining resource from this root. So I would argue that only a renovation of the Tradition can save us in the present and in the future. The argument is not conservative; it is radical. Only by tapping resources from the moral root of our heritage can we understand reality, particularly in its most enigmatic realm: human health and disease.

The book, in other words, seeks to discern the heuristic value of the Tradition. By this I do not mean some past structure of meaning from which we then attempt to construe normative significance. There is, I believe, a sense of the good perceptible to reason and conscience, a quality of the historical and existential experience which bears a message to us as to what is right, what is appropriate or fitting, what is wholesome. There is, I contend, an inherited normative understanding of what health and illness mean in the human experience. The argument is an extension of the earlier thesis which argued that the good will be self-evident if we remember our tradition, probe our conscience and common sense, and weigh the future. Only a normative value and vision can serve to guide us in the decisions we must make regarding our generativity, our suffering, our disease and well being, our death.

The book is not merely an intellectual exercise. It is written as a diary of a personal struggle. I work day by day in one of the world's great centers of medicine in Houston, a tertiary care center where sick people come as a last resort. As traditional treatment modalities have failed, here the glimmer of hope leads desperate families to try the newest procedure, often costly and accompanied by harsh side effects, when the risks frequently counteract the benefits. "What is for the patient's good?" is a question that today requires more than technical judgments. Discernments of meaning and value are required, together with sound scientific analyses. In health care centers today, we are forced to do reflective medicine and constructive theology. Indeed, the two inquiries merge.

Three urgent reasons compel the present study. First, the emerging scientific mood requires an increasingly complex and broad range of factors to explain nature's process. Secondly, although health and disease are conceived and interpreted empirically and technically in the scientific world, in the common wisdom of people, religion still provides the salience by which these experiences are valued and disvalued. This is not an Archie Bunker–type argument contending that the divinity of Jesus is proved by the fact that people around the world celebrate Christmas. Rather, it is recognition that *consensus fidelium*, general moral wisdom, always provides the surest ethical norm. Finally, there is the necessity to move toward a better ethical knowledge and a sharpened moral consciousness. The particular issues we must now face—not only the interventions we now have power to make along the life-cycle but the challenges of fashioning human nature and remaking human beings—demand normative insights that we have never before possessed. We need to get our normative image of people in focus before we set out to change their nature.

Evidence from the sciences, ranging from astrophysics and cosmology to cell biophysics and genetics, continues to expand the narrow explanation of the nature of things that characterized nineteenth-century modes of knowing. Because of the work of Planck, Einstein, and Heisenberg in physics and Freud, Jung, and Adler in the behavioral sciences, mechanistic, reductionistic understandings of cause and effect no longer prevail. New dimensions of depth, complexity, and mystery replace older simplifications in explanations of what constitutes human beings and their activity.

In the modern world, medicine especially has capitulated to positivism, denying dimensions of spirit and value. This was necessary; the roots of magic and superstition from which medicine and psychotherapy emerged demanded a dramatic break. Now the positive values of the legacy need to be recovered lest we continue to distort healing into technical manipulation, setting in motion internal contradictions in health care and doing harm in the name of healing. We need again to be touched by infinite meaning so that our mundane tasks can be borne with courage.

It is patients—those who have been the beneficiaries and victims of biomedical knowledge and technology—who have forced open again the sense of depth. People who are growing and being healed, as well as those who, in the process of becom-

ing whole, endure suffering and death, teach us that health
and disease are spiritual and moral experiences. Deep currents
of meaning are part of illness and healing. Each insight of
value in this book has been reached in a crucible of hope and
pain. Each teacher has been a sufferer, a patient.

Despite the way the laity has been fascinated with the
technological age, religious ideas continue to structure the way
we comprehend well-being and illness.[6] Not only the enduring
power of folk medicine but also empirical data attest to this
fact. The clinical experience of educated, nonsuperstitious
persons is to interpret health and illness theologically. Even the
so-called "secularized" individual often casts the experience of
illness and healing in terms of judgment, guilt, responsibility,
reorientation, and salvation. I propose that these perceptions
are not anxiety-induced distortions but true reading of the nature of reality. We come to our senses in illness. It is my conviction that theological discernments of the meanings of health
and disease will enrich our scientific understanding of, as well
as our community response to, these tragic and blissful tones of
our life.

Finally, the times demand such analysis because of ethical
quandries inherent in our scientific progress. Concerns of
biomedical ethics pervade the medical and popular literature.
Those moralists leading the inquiry insist that we can no longer
produce instant occasional wisdom for problem after problem,
such as genetics, abortion, transplantation, behavior modification, and death. We must first probe the foundation questions.
Both philosophical and theological ethicists know that we must
inquire after a basic philosophy of medicine or a theology of
health and disease before the specific "problem centered"
guidelines can be developed.

In summary, two present factors render the Experiment
wanting and call us to recover the truth and value of the Tradition. First, new knowledge about the onset and progression of

illness suggests that a wholistic, psychosomatic, organically complex process model, not the mechanistic model of the Experiment, better explains health and illness. Secondly, the therapeutic encounter between healer and patient discloses how complex a process is the cause and progression of disease. Moral and spiritual dimensions as well as life-style interplay with physical causes. The healer is forced to the wholistic view no matter how desirable a simplistic, specific etiology would be. In order for there to be a true and total conception of what health and disease are, we must synthesize into an interrelated whole the insights gained from natural and supernatural science.

When Albert Schweitzer first arrived in Lambarene and stood at the edge of the primeval forest, he wrote of an ethical vision that transcended the rational. Today we stand at such a threshold. Schweitzer spoke of the necessity for a "better knowledge," a finely honed conscience, that alone can guide at the edge of an unknown both foreboding and enticing. The spirit of Schweitzer provides a controlling mood for this study. It remains to be seen whether our civilization, the first in world history to exert dominion over nature's caprice in the realm of disease, a civilization blessed with substance and health, can discover with Cicero that we are all dying caring for the dying and are obliged, therefore, to fashion a new theology of health and disease as the foundation for a new ethics of compassion. Though our new orientation cannot have the paternalism of Schweitzer's world view, it desperately needs his sense of mutuality and respect for life and health.

Today we are possessed with a passion, some say a madness, for perfection and technical defeat of the forces that inflict disease and death. From another vantage point, this can be seen as a yearning for well-being, a desire to have healthy offspring, a hope for relative health during our precarious pilgrimage, a quest to approximate our earthly existence more closely to the Kingdom of God. While we need to be sustained by this natural and transcending vision, we also need to graciously accept those boundaries which, when considered generationally, cosmically, and under the purview of eternity, are blessings. Maintaining the delicate tension between ascendency and acceptance seems to be one of the most crucial tasks facing us.

In words that can serve as a touchstone for this inquiry, Galen, the epitome of Greco-Roman medical wisdom, said: "It would be vain to expect to see living beings formed of the blood of menstrous women and the semen viril, who will not die, will never feel pain, or will move perpetually, or will shine like the sun."[7]

The glory of humanity is found not in the ability to overcome its limitations but in the ability to transform flaw into strength, draw out the purposive from the absurd, meet the Eternal in the time-bound. In growth, suffering, and death we fashion this crowning achievement.

Here follows an exercise in theology and medical ethics. Surely one of the most illuminating sources of theological insight, that is, who God is and what he is doing, is human experience, especially that experience chastened by health and illness. Thus this book seeks to help the religious community fashion its theological understanding of life in the modern world. It is also a constructive critique of modern medicine and a positive commendation of a different, more wholesome, approach. Just a small step forward from either side will have made the effort well worthwhile.

II

The Tradition

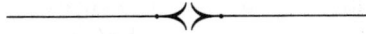

———————◇———————

An' I've made foot mats out'n corn shucks—t'wipe yer feet
on. That's easy, an' that's th' prettiest work! They make th'
best foot mats. I ain't made none since m' hand's paralyzed.
I reckon God just didn't intend fer me t'work my hand!
                                          —AUNT ARIE. *The Foxfire Book I* [1]

Primitive peoples seem to accept as a reasonable explanation of
their fate that human life is under the simultaneous influence of
supernatural as well as natural forces. They are prone to trace their
misfortunes and diseases to the evil doings of ghosts, witches and
other demonic powers; but they also know from experience that the
body and mind are directly affected by the elementary forces of
nature that they can perceive with their senses. In fact, this dual
attitude is not peculiar to primitive people. Even in the most sophis-
ticated communities, belief in mysterious influences still coexists
with the knowledge derived from rational philosophy and science.
Lovers and poets are not the only ones to acknowledge that
springtime awakens the senses, autumn engenders melancholy,
and the stars inspire suprarational dreams. [2]

René Dubos thus summarizes the heart of the primitive
Tradition as it bears on our understanding of our place in
nature as well as our perception of the forces that interplay to
determine our health and well-being. People perceive themselves as both free and determined, both acting and acted
upon. They understand certain things that happen to them;
other things remain mysterious or "yet to be understood."

A certain range of experience is always in transition from the realm of mystery to the realm of comprehension. This then becomes experience that can no longer be fatalistically accepted. It becomes the kind of knowledge that draws out the will to understand and control.

Often people will attribute to divine cause the scourge whose source is not understood. This view of divine providence is usually provisional, however. When Cotton Mather decided to advocate smallpox vaccination in Massachusetts, he did not abandon his belief that God was "the commander of disease." Rather than taking a posture of resignation, he saw disease as a force to challenge human ingenuity to do something about it. Though the Creator allows pain to infiltrate the creation, he stands with us for health against disease and disorder. Though disease and death are inimical to life, they are necessary. In life and death, health and illness, God is our companion.

Morris Leikind, writing on colonial epidemic diseases, describes the response of New England to the third great plague and continues with a poem that expresses the tentativeness of the providential theodicy.

The throat distemper as it was called was a complex matter. It actually consisted of three separate epidemics—one of scarlet fever and two of diphtheria. Because of inaccurate diagnosis and inadequate clinical differentiation the diseases were confused and associated under a common name. The epidemic which seems to be connected with Kingston, New Hampshire, began in 1735 and was actually a small part of a widespread involvement of the whole of New England. In a period of five years, 5,000 persons died, mostly children and young people. A most curious fact is the comparative absence of public hysteria in the face of such a catastrophe. With two, often three, and even six and seven children in a family being carried off within a few days, the tragedy was often regarded as an act of God and accepted with an unquestioning faith.

The cause of the epidemic in those pre-microbial days was, of
course, unknown, and even the doctors admitted their helpless-
ness. A contemporary poem tells us:

> The Doctor's Art, can find no part,
>   nor Cure for this Distemper;
> By Physic long, nor Cordials strong,
>   they cannot find the Center.
>
> It is unknown to any one
>   and all the Doctors skill,
> To cure this Plague, or to engage
>   to cure it at their will.
>
> They're in the dark, in every part,
>   and cannot find it out,
> From whence it strikes, and where it
>   lights they cannot point it out.
>
> If we should call the Doctors all
>   and let them all engage,
> We cannot find in any kind that
>   they can cure this Plague.
>
> Let's search the Cause, 'tis breach of Laws,
>   that punishes for Sin,
> That brings down Plagues in every Age,
>   as it has ever been.
>
> Ungrateful Sins have ever been
>   most odious in God's Sight
> Then let's repent with one consent,
>   and pray both Day and Night.[3]

In this chapter we will survey that interpretation of reality
that will be called the Tradition. This world view, common to

all pre-modern cultures, has an image of man in nature as microcosm, a view of disease as announcement, and a vision of healing as cleansing and restoration.

MAN AS MICROCOSM

In the traditional understanding, man pictures himself as integral to all nature, a microcosm of the great drama unfolding in the cosmos. This microcosmic self-understanding is common to the several interpretations of the meaning of health and disease that constitute what we will call the Tradition. It is seen in primitive medicine and its lingerings in modern folk medicine. It constitutes the essence of Greek medical wisdom. It is found in the religiomedical perceptions of Judaism and Christianity.

Primitive peoples experience disease in a twofold manner. On the one hand they see that life is part of the great cycle of nature and that human beings are subject to the same forces of decay and death that prevail in the cosmos. The great murals on the walls of tombs and temples from the pre-Classical period in Egypt depict rich concepts of interrelation and interdependence. Man, woman, and child are pictured as an organic part of nature, with the animals, plants, and stars each placed so as to constitute a harmonious whole. The divine sun irradiates the portrait. In the famed fifth-century mosaics at Ravenna, the same cosmic drama is depicted. Christ, the good shepherd or *Pantokrator*, oversees the whole creation with blue skies and seas, trees, birds, and people. All have their place in nature, all belong together, fulfilling one another's being through interdependence. In both of these works not only do nature's rhythms ebb and flow within human beings, but they picture themselves as a mirror which reflects the broader cosmic image, beings within whom the broader cosmic story is enacted.

Flaws and illness, healing and growth, destruction and disease all contribute to the coloration of nature's panorama; and as microcosmic symbols of reality, they form the bittersweetness of existence.

In Navajo thought, the basic disposition of a person is considered to be shaped by the cosmic winds and rays. The winds come into a person at birth and determine a "soul without meanness" or a "mean soul." A person's place in relation to the sun determines whether he or she is a "sunwise soul," or a "sunward soul" who will destroy things, hurt people, and so forth.[4]

The primitive peoples also see such processes and events as contradictions to nature's benevolence. They are negations of what should be. They constitute a fabric of evil that is inimical to human desire and what is taken to be a deeper cosmic purpose. Many primitive peoples develop dualistic views of nature, wherein demonic forces vie with good and natural energies for dominance in human beings. Out of this spirit, ancient people formed systems of magic and witchcraft which are the other side of the primitive reaction to disease and suffering.

It must be noted that magic and superstition are an advance, not a retardation, in moral development. They are the first expressions of human unwillingness to be passive against fate, a seeking to manipulate and control. In this sense, they are a precursor of a desire to change reality and not just accept it.

This duality of response—resignation and resistance, acquiescence and active control—remains the perennial ambivalence of the fully human response. The graceful acceptance of disease and death shapes the central disposition of the traditional sense. The resignation element of the Tradition cannot be accepted. Reaction to it spurs investigation and therapeutic intervention and is the formative impulse of what will be called the Experiment. Both moods interplay in the suggested synthesis that we will call the Renovation.

The microcosmic view considers that people are affected by natural and supernatural forces. The gods and demons traffic with them. History is replete with examples where disease is seen to be caused by demons. From primitive tribal superstitions to the equally superstitious and even more dangerous etiological theories of the Puritans in early Massachusetts, we find that cultural periods characterized by religious intensity tend to project the enigma of disease causation on to alien powers and beings. Ancient Near Eastern societies at the time of Christ interpreted onsets of illness and healing in this way. The Christian Church and modern societies living in its legacy have great difficulty understanding this mentality. The narrative in the gospel of Matthew, for example, is punctuated with healing events from beginning to end. Modern people, proud of their newly liberated scientific intellect, must either write the accounts off as literary fantasy or demythologize the stories to fit the new heavenless flat world.

I will suggest later in this chapter why such repudiation is unnecessary and how enduring validity can be found in the demonic interpretation of disease as well as the attribution of healing to the divine power.

The Navajos express another microcosmic view of human life that bears on understandings of disease and healing. Human beings are windows of earth and sky. The Great Spirit stands over life, sustaining their beings by the natural world made for their sustenance. To be sick is to be momentarily torn out of the divine and human fabric which nurtures life and health. The Navajo healing rite begins with two stages of purification and prayer for recovery. Then the ritual seeks to reestablish the alienated and ostracized individual in the divine-human community. To be reintegrated into the life of the holy people (sickness has broken this identity), the sufferer is laid on a mural depicting the community, which is painted in the sand,

and is pressed down until the body pattern is imprinted on the sand picture. The individual is thereby accepted again into the society, into the fabric of communal life, and the mural is again complete. The microcosm takes its place again within the macrocosm. A bodily identification of the human with the divine is achieved.[5]

The University of Oregon Health Sciences Center is actively searching for an Indian medicine man to join a mental health project. Part of a congressional program which seeks to apply the insights of folk healing traditions among blacks, Mexican-Americans, Asian-Americans and native Americans, the project reflects a new openness of spirit, willing to retain the wisdom of these venerable traditions.

There is also enduring value in other primitive notions of human beings as microcosm. If we are to salvage the genius of this conception, the demonic view of health and disease today must undergo rigorous reformation. It can, and indeed must, be reincorporated into our modern scientific understanding. What Walter Lipmann called the "acids of modernity" should be allowed to fully erode the unnatural, the dehumanizing, the freedom-negating encrustations on the demonic etiology of disease. But the genius of the primitive notion is what is transmitted in Socrates' sense of the *daimon*—a mediation which conveys the significance of that which is beyond human beings and inimical to their purpose. The demon is at once accepted and challenged. This view of the demonic is well worth our examination and acceptance. Perhaps the recovery of this concept would engender a wholistic, natural sense of the meaning of health and disease and rescue us from the further human ravages of a narrow scientific-technical view.

A former president of the Royal College of Physicians has argued that much science and technology of value are present in primitive medicine. "That primitive belief that the spiritual world is the one source of health has a positive lesson for our own day."[6] What are some examples of the enduring insights of primitive peoples regarding health and disease?

The medical ministrations of the traditional cultures serve as an example. In a graduation address to Baylor College of Medicine, Eugene Stead, a renowned professor of internal medicine, extolled the wisdom of the multifaceted Chinese system of health care, which combines folk traditions along with the strengths of scientific medicine. Similarly, Douglas Guthrie addressed the Royal Society of Medicine, taking note of the strengths of the "supernatural" approach of the African medicine man.

> He proceeds with his diagnosis, not in order to give the disease a name and apply appropriate treatment, but in order to ascertain its cause and remove it. The method is based on the belief that something has entered the patient's body, or something has been extracted from the patient's body. The invader may be an evil spirit . . . or it may be a material intrusion. . . . This idea of some simple particle projected into the body and causing disease is an ancient belief which is really quite rational.[7]

Here we see the positive value of the primitive microcosmic view of humanity. Disease ensues when something alien enters in or something vital goes out of the person. Disease is disruption of the rhythmic flow of the resources of life from organism to organism. When the cycles of life from air, land, and water flow into and through us, we are well. The tubercle bacillus has a benign effect in nature until it finds a home in weakened, predisposed people, where it multiplies out of proportion. The natural flora and fauna present in our intestines have a positive effect until breakdown occurs when they fracture the constraints of the customarily resistant body. The primitive picture of the microcosm has a perennial validity.

A further enduring insight of primitive medicine is the notion that sick people perceive their plight with a burden of guilt and accept healing and restoration as gift and blessing. Primitive people sense that they have offended the divine order of things when they become ill. Their situation is therefore not accidental. They are responsible for and morally involved in the dynamics of suffering and healing. As a microcosm of nature and supernature, they do not see themselves as hapless victims of blind processes; they are acting and acted upon. They therefore must be morally engaged in what is happening even in the midst of illness. An authority on African medicine has stated:

> Health of body and of mind are so related that although the so-called medicine man may be deficient in physical science, his function as a soul-doctor has to be treated as on the whole salutary given the psychological condition of his patients. . . . As for his views about disease, this is normally treated as a sort of spiritual visitation, the result of an enemy's spells on the patient's own sinfulness; so that his cure correspondingly takes the form of an exorcism designed to dispel fear and restore confidence. Accidentally, however, many of such methods of expelling evil by means of blood-letting, purging, trephining and so on have a physical no less than a moral effect.[8]

For all the difficulty this view poses for any metaphysics, it must be stated that modern people, like the ancients, often perceive disease and health in this way. Their psychic and emotional response often casts experiences into this framework. It seems to me that the fact that we experience illness and recovery in terms of guilt and grace and that modern people perceive these experiences in the same way as primitive people proves that Freud was mistaken when he interpreted guilt and grace as distortions growing out of our cosmic anxiety. Is it possible that the enduring quality of these perceptions provides evidence for the *meta*physical and *super*natural dimensions of the physical and natural phenomena of disease and health?

A brief glimpse at the microcosmic view in the medicine of ancient and modern China will illustrate this perception of nature and supernature as continuous. The genius of the ancient medical tradition apparently is still vibrant in the intellectual system and the practical delivery mechanism of modern Chinese medicine. Here again, human life is seen as a microcosm of heaven and earth. People carry within themselves the dialectic and tension that exist in external reality. In the realm of psychology and physiology, life is characterized by the generation of opposites and tensions. The Yin and Yang, fundamental energies in reality, interplay in the organism as well as in the external world. The dynamics of physical and mental process, particularly the twelve channels that hold vital balance in the body, are activated by Yin and Yang, growth and disintegration, healing and tearing, living and dying.

> Health is pictured as equilibrium or balancing of these tensions. . . . The harmony of opposites; of rhythm between the active and passive, the creative and receptive, between motion and repose . . . health is achieved by the adjustment of [the] whole being, body and spirit, to the creative forces of the universe.[9]

The People's Republic of China has fashioned today what can only be called a remarkable health care system. Each person sees himself or herself as an essential part of the whole. Acupuncture, barefoot doctoring, and psychological conditioning are expressions of an advanced system that is undergirded by the old metaphysics. Those who have visited China under recent exchange programs have returned lauding the way in which a self-care, preventive medicine and health delivery system has been fashioned to serve 800 million people.

The cynic will say that the Communist brainwashing has de-
stroyed individualism so that people see themselves as expend-
able for the whole. A more generous view would honor the
remarkable progress and appreciate the sense in which all individuals play a creative part in the communal solidarity. In
either case, the traditional microcosmic notion is operative.

Man is microcosm in a completely different sense to the
Hebrews. The Old Testament does not contain a systematic
view of nature or anthropology. Its story is that of the saving
acts of God. The Old Testament chronicles the history of a
people who sensed a divine investiture and a divine beckoning
in their common life. Yaweh had drawn near to dwell in them
and with them. They are the image of God. God has carved his
form into their being. They are vessels—their maker fashions
their shape as with a clay vase and pours life or breath into that
form—so they are microcosmic not so much of nature as of
supernature. Their flesh does not incarnate an immortal soul
nor do they hold within them a divine spark. They are divinely
constituted. Their being is a picture of God. Man is a microcosm in that the spiritual and moral reality of God is continuous with human life. People are spiritual beings; that is, they
have access to realms of reality that transcend time and space.
The quality of eternity has a claim on their life. Their being can
entertain or frustrate the spirit of God. In the midst of death,
they can be caught up in *zoen aionion* (life eternal.)

A moral impulse also moves through humanity. Human beings are drawn into levels of virtue and love because God is
righteous. Because of this microcosmic sense of their nature
and destiny, the Jews regard disease and health as morally and
spiritually conditioned. Sickness is both punishment for sin
and atonement for guilt. It thus becomes an experience with
repenting and redeeming quality. The lasting significance of
this strain in our Tradition is that it repudiates the notion that
disease is blind, purposeless happenstance. Hebrew faith holds

that nothing afflicts creatures of God if he himself has not censured them. Every evil that befalls humanity must pass his scrutiny. His will takes every event, however tragic, to its redeeming and healing consummation.

The Hippocratic and broader Greek understanding, also microcosmic, rounds out my consideration of the traditional concept of the human in nature. Although the seeds for experimental scientific medicine are present in the Hippocratic tradition, the essence of the mood is humanistic. Physicians and philosophers in the spirit of Hippocrates were much like the students of Plato and Aristotle. They were impatient with spiritualized explanations of natural phenomena when the only justification for such explanations was the absence of empirical verification. Epilepsy was no more a "holy" disease than any other. They said, "Why do things happen? Let us inquire, question our assumptions and prejudices, test explanations against the evidence. Finally, let us decide and act, with full trust in the divine foreground and background of nature." This was the spirit and is the enduring significance of Greek medicine.

The Greek sense of human life as microcosm is the anthropology undergirding her intellectual system.Nature is like man, they said; yes, even supernature: the gods are like men. Greeks thus felt at home in nature. Nature was stripped of its demonic terror. Harmony was sought between man, nature, and the gods. The gods pitied man, played with him, often capriciously, but most often lovingly. For all the ways his life was continuous with nature and the gods, the fundamental tragic discontinuity remained: man was mortal. He could yearn for immortality; like Prometheus he could steal the divine fire; but all hubristic overshooting of bounds was doomed. Resignation, courage, acceptance of fate and boundaries were dispositions that led to harmony and peace. *Mens sana in corpore sano*: an intact and stable mind within a beautiful body; this was microcosmic health.

This Greek sense of reality, which saw continuities between the human mind and the processes of cause and effect in nature, gradually developed a system of belief in the laws, regularities, and predictabilities of nature. Natural modes of explanation do not, of course, answer the "why" questions of health and disease. They do, however, further our comprehension of how sickness and health unfold.

The Greek sense of microcosm also gave rise to a great flaw in the Tradition. When health was seen as harmony with the rhythms and perfections of nature, dysrhythms and imperfections were seen as inferior states. The sick person was devalued and often disregarded, as were the weak and disabled. Compassion and pity for suffering humanity, as Nietzsche reminded us centuries later, were, for the Greeks, dangerous, pathetic, and sentimental virtues.

Finally, the mythic structure that has most deeply shaped our traditional culture as it ponders the mystery of disease and health is the biblical story which is received at the axis times where Hebrew meets Greek culture. The power of these symbols continues to pervade our culture and determine the ways we look at and respond to these experiences.

The story can be divided into four chapters. In origin and intention, the world is a haven for human fulfillment as the friend and partner of God. Abundant provision is made for our need. Life is blissful. There is no disease, no death. We are possessed with the glory and risk of freedom. We are free to pursue or contradict our character, our purpose, our happiness. A cleavage opens when we depart from what we should and could be in association with our Maker and our fellows. We know good and evil and choose the latter.

The ascent or fall of humanity introduces tension, anxiety, and strife into our existence and the common life. Not only is the self-relation and fellowship with God shattered, but an enmity within nature is set in motion. Forces of disease, destruction, and death are let loose in the world. While much pain in the direct consequence of our misuse of freedom, fraternal malice, and lust for destruction, a total disharmony is introduced and the cosmic song becomes discordant.

But God cares and will not abandon his handiwork or give up on his friend. A redemptive purpose ensues wherein the very tension initiated in willfulness and rebellion becomes the yearning force that will carry the creation forward toward its consummate purpose. Disease and death become both the sting of a poisoned creation and the image of hope of a world that is coming. Two impulses characterize human life in this interim time. One attitude is anger at being expelled from paradise; the other seeks to patiently build the awaited Kingdom. Both energies are technological and creative. They attempt to insulate and enhance our tragic existence. We become scientist and therapist. Our imagination and action can be motivated by indignation or cooperation. Our work either destroys or heals. Disease, like physical pain, becomes the sign that mending is going on and redemption is fashioning renewed creation. The redeemer is a chosen people, the Messiah, the incorporated body through which salvation and healing are given to the creation. In the power of this personalized saving spirit, health is breathed into life.

The final chapter of the story speaks of a moment that is coming, assured by tangible anticipations. A state of affairs will develop or appear wherein the flaws will be remedied, rough places explained and planed, and all life won back to its intention. In brokenness, sickness, and death, our life is bound to the constraints of the story's beginning. In health, healing, salvation, and eternal life, we are allowed to foretaste the consummation of the story.

In summary, the Tradition has seen human beings as fragments, reflections, microcosms of the broader and profounder reality, not different and discontinuous. By contrast, man is not microcosm in the Experiment; he is master over nature. The Tradition distills to the essence that human beings, though

finite, participate in the infinite. Our life intersects and is inter-
sected by the reality of God and the Realm of nature. We are
indeed both godlike and animal (a little lower than the angels);
both matter and spirit. Our destiny, including those forces that
affect us in both wholesome and disturbing ways, is in many
senses conditioned by the divine and natural fabric which is the
setting of our life. Now we must examine the meaning that
health and disease assume against this world picture.

DISEASE AS MESSAGE

"I am dying," a gracious and godly old woman told me,
"because I am a sinner." Her words at first were disturbing.
They were difficult for me to understand because I am a child
of the Experiment. This causal linking of sin and sickness
smacks of an age of witchcraft, of repression and judgment
that we had hoped was far behind us. Yet on deeper reflection,
her words had a freshness, a power, a sense of truth.

At the heart of the Tradition we find the view that sickness
and death prevail in the natural and human world because
something has gone wrong. The word *pain* itself implies these
meanings. The word is derived from the Latin root *Poena*,
punishment, and ultimately from the Sanskrit root *Pu,* purification.

In this section I will examine the traditional view that finds in
disease chastising or cathartic meaning. I will also consider the
correlative notion that health implies righteousness. The purpose will be to see in what ways, if any, these understandings
remain valid. Again, I will examine several cultural streams
that flow within the Tradition. Particular attention will be
given to Judaism and Christianity, with only occasional insights
drawn from primitive and folk traditions and the Greeks.

The people of the Old and New Covenant come to understand health and disease in a peculiar way. At the simplest level,
it is acknowledged that much disease and suffering will be

removed if people seek righteousness and obey the Law of God. The Decalogue and its elaborations within the Pentateuch point to the fact that if human beings love themselves and their neighbors with all the strength of heart, mind, and will, they will not be inflicted with the measure of evil that will be their lot if misdirection, idolatry, and sin control their lives. If sanitary and dietary regulations are heeded; if cleanliness, faithfulness, and love abound within the community, individuals and the society will be well.[10]

This is not to say that sickness, suffering, and death will be obliterated. These deeper reaches of the enigma of human frailty will prevail. Even the righteous will suffer and die. Since Job and the Psalmist, the perplexing theological quandary remains; even the righteous suffer. A primary meaning of the story of Job is that pain is not necessarily punishment, nor is prosperity necessarily reward.

The people of Israel are quarantined from certain diseases if life remains obedient to the divine will. S. J. McMillen's *None of These Diseases* points to the way this divine immunization will take place if the laws of circumcision, diet, cleanliness, and life-style are followed.[11] Yet disease and mortality as unalterable conditions of life will still afflict even obedient people.

In his monumental *Ancient Judaism*,[12] Max Weber discusses the way that this faith is different from the other ancient religions in the accent placed on a living moral tradition. The profound covenant was elaborated in the Levitical code to express a total way of life. Within this law, righteousness, health, and soul care were safeguarded and sustained. It is important to note the radically novel way in which moral guidance, mental health, and total well-being are integrated in this understanding.

In late Judaism, eschatological and messianic consciousness came to influence piety and literature, and the theme of sickness and suffering takes on redemptive meaning. It is this religious faith, along with the faith of primitive Christianity that it yields, that lends the Tradition its loftiest insights on health and disease.

The central element of biblical faith that brings meaning to disease is the notion of the nature of God. In this theology and worship, God himself, though sovereign and immutable, is a being who can be spoken of as a loving, caring, yearning, pain-bearing savior. God in the Hebrew scripture is a pathetic being; he feels for and with humanity. He heals; he saves. Two passages from the exilic period stand out; the Royal Servant is seen in grotesque leprous visage:

> He has no form or loveliness; that we should look at him, and no beauty that we should be attracted to him. He was despised and rejected by men; a man of sorrows, familiar with sickness; and as one from whom men turn their heads he was despised and we esteemed him not.

> He has borne our diseases and carried out sorrows . . . with his pain we are healed (Isaiah 53:2–4).

Psychiatrists Price Cobbs and William H. Grier report the following case in their study *Black Rage*.

> The Negro man of 80 told a story. He was 12 and a playmate was tied in a cage waiting to be taken away and lynched . . . (the shackled boy stood accused of raping a white woman.)
> The old man recalled the fright which caused him to run away the next day. From that time on he never knew a home. His years were spent roaming about the country. He became an itinerant preacher, forever invoking God, but always too terrified to return to his place of birth. When asked why, he would reply: "The white folks down there are too mean."
> For most of his life he was tormented by memories. Every place he stopped, he soon became frightened and moved on. Sometimes in the middle of a sermon he would cry out: "How could they do that to a boy?"[13]

Bubba died of malignant melanoma at the hospital which adjoins our Institute. He was a young man, in the flowering of his vocation, splendidly trained, a minister and theological professor, when a mole appeared on the back of his leg. A careless oversight, a bungled diagnosis; finally, a belated excision and a positive biopsy ensued. Bubba was preaching a mission when the truth hit. He felt something radiating up from the mole into a lymph node. He knew he was dead. Although dread swept over him, he also related a deep pervasive sense of calm. Then followed months of intermittent, then fulltime, hospitalization, finally that admission from which there would be no return. He carefully chose his physician. The energy of hope and the yearning to live prompted him to come to an advanced medical center and work with a distinguished physician who was advancing frontiers of treatment. He also selected his surgeon-oncologist on the basis of his writings, which showed heightened and somewhat exceptional sensitivity to the psychodynamic dimensions of catastrophic illness. He forced his physician to be just that: one who would move with him as a partner into those profound transactions of hope and fear, radical treatment and restraint—one who would help him maximally relish the life that remained and courageously go to meet death. He would not allow his doctor to withdraw. He asked all who accompanied him on this last adventure to remain open and honest—retaining, as he did, that earthy sense of humor that Dostoevsky found to be the essence of humanness and humility. He taught all who knew him the gracious sense of mingled terror, mystery, and comfort that is in the profound biblical sense of the meaning of disease.

Memorial services were held in cities around the country— his home town, his schools, towns where he had served as pastor. As he had wished, the text for meditation was John 13. Jesus, on the eve of his death, surrounded by the threat of violence, the foreboding of the unknown, amid a rush of events absurdly senseless, took the basin and the towel, knelt and washed the feet of his friends.

For Bubba, this Last Supper act became the paradigm of a human response to disease and death, the only way that the Christian could imbue this trauma with meaning. There is no easy rhyme or reason to our being and destiny in this world. Life is cruciform; and the important thing is that our being is faithful as it is embodied in life together. In this precipitous night, like that night of nights, we can only kneel and serve one another. In suffering and in death, Bubba witnessed to the truth of life's deepest paradox: "In dying we live."

As Jesus died on the cross, he cried in dereliction: "Why hast thou forsaken me?" He is recalling the ancient servant cry in Psalm 22. The question is, as theologian Jürgen Moltmann argues, the root question of all theology. It is also the question of the atheistic rebellion against God.[14] It is surely the fundamental question of any theological treatment of the meaning of health and disease. The deepest meaning we can derive is that, in some profound sense, God bears and shares our pain and disease. In some mysterious sense, suffering draws us to the heart of the meaning of reality. Therefore, disease in Judeo-Christian thought is not only a contradiction but an experience that can be received as meaning, as prophesy, as voice of God, as revelation. Equilibrium and continuity are shattered, composure is shaken. Yet life is fractured open as new possibilities, both destructive and creative, present themselves.

Likewise, the Tradition in general perceives disease as warning. Primitive people see disease as an intruder into personal wholeness, communal solidarity, and cosmic order. The Greeks saw illness as disequilibrium, imbalance, or discoloration.

Our Christian moral and spiritual tradition sees illness as the consequence of sin and the opportunity for salvation. It is an evil and chaotic disturbance of what should be, the consequence of rebellion in the creation. Yet the malignancy of disease in this tradition is not merely imbalance and disorder. Illness is not a blind, furious, chaotic force that disturbs the composition and intention of nature. It is not the malicious working of some ultimate Being seeking to create fear and receive propitiation. It is crisis in the sense that the rupture discloses something and can be purposive. Let us examine this sense of the meaning of health and disease by first examining the notion that disease is a message. We will then consider the relationship of sin and sickness, and finally the meaning of illness as message.

Behind the view of disease as message is a view of God, humanity, the world that must be understood. God is making the creation into the kind of responding organism that he designs it to be. Human freedom has been misused, in that we have gravitated away from God and have let loose impediments to his will on the earth. His purpose is wholeness, health, growth, and happiness. He has set us within families and nations on an abundant and resourceful earth. The apocryphal book of the Wisdom of Solomon (1:7, 12–16) speaks of the health God intends for his creation.

> The Spirit of the Lord filleth the World. . . . Seek not death in the error of your life and pull not upon yourselves destruction with the works of your hands. For God made not death; neither hath He pleasure in the destruction of the living. For He created all things that they might have their being; and the generations of the world were healthful; and there is no poison of destruction on them, nor the Kingdom of Death upon the earth: [for righteousness is immortal]. But ungodly men with their works and words called it to them.

Cardinal Newman has said we are not merely imperfect creatures who need to be improved; we are rebels who need to lay down our arms. Part of the terror of the pain that throbs in the heart of the universe is the tortuous task of tearing our will from its locus in rebellion and restoring it to God—its true home. C. S. Lewis, much in the spirit of Dostoevsky, claims that we suffer intensely as humans because of the discrepancy between what we are and what we know we ought to be and could be. Health and disease are, by definition, ethical and eschatological questions. We bring meaning to our physical pain, suffering, and death that symbolize our more basic *meta*physical or spiritual disease.

We feel at dis-ease spiritually because we trust that the world is moving more toward its divine destiny and that we too are in process of becoming new creatures. Freedom is painful. Profound choices are difficult. To be mature is extremely threatening. Yet we know that the world is ordered proleptically and that nature is eschatologically tempered. That is, our own being, indeed the whole creation of which we are a part, groans and yearns toward newness and perfection. Expectation of hope draws us on from the present incompleteness, imperfection, disease, and sorrow toward that future where these wounds are healed. This is why we experience disease as problematic. Emil Fackenheim has written:

> Divine providence is human freedom and consists of its progressive realization. Meaning in history lies in its forward direction—one in which human freedom raises itself ever higher toward Divinity, and evil comes closer to being conquered.[15]

The experience of pain is heightened as phylogenetic evolution branches upward into the human species. Rocks and trees, though subject to the same physical processes of destruction, genetically conditioned loads, and other deteriorative processes, are not seen to be caught up in tragic process. Though pain in the animals remains a profound enigma, we do not interpret this as evil. In human beings, however, disease and suffering are given meaning. The *why* is a uniquely human

probe. It signals the fact that people must seek to make sense
out of what happens to them.

The Judeo-Christian sense that God is Creator—that he
wills our well-being and salvation, that he has decisively entered our history and shared the tragedy of our existence—
evokes an interpretation of health and disease as a message.
The first important sense in which we can speak of illness as a
voice is that there is a discrepancy between what we are and
what we might be. A disharmony exists, a discord that seeks
resolution. The state of health or well-being is thus a precondi-
tion of any sense of what disease is. Kaspar Naegele, in an
important book on healing, has spoken of the difficulty of
talking about health as a positive quality.

> It is a condition necessary for the realization of two of our regnant
> values: mastery of the world and fun. Yet as a desired end health is
> both ubiquitous and empty. One is never without it, but it is never
> clear what one possesses in having it.[16]

Illness is a voice in two senses. First, it is experience that
makes us aware of how far we are from health. In the words of
the Book of Common Prayer, we know "there is no health in
us." Secondly, the voice of illness beckons us to become our
true self. The summer before last, after a day's work and
shower, I discovered that my body was covered with red
patches. My immediate response was terror. I remembered a
dear friend who, the summer before, had returned from vacation with such a rash, soon discovered she had an acute form of
lymphocitic leukemia, and was dead in two months. After the
initial fright I found my response to be one of examining criti-
cally my active sense of what was important, reaffirming what I
really valued as I searched my heart, and vowing to get
priorities straight. I resolved that time was infinitely precious
and that each moment should be fully claimed in its significance. My relationship to and vocation under God surfaced

with vivid reality. The desire rose to love and respond to my children and wife more sensitively. Fortunately, or unfortunately as the case may be, the rash left. The next day came and, as I was convinced again of my own immortality, the more routine desensitization took over.

Although Riese sees this kind of experience as a "trivial fact," it would seem to be an insight of monumental significance into human nature.

> Man may experience through pain a complete change in his mode of existence. It is not a philosophical statement but almost a trivial fact that pain and suffering induce a conscious experience of limitation and weakness. Thus, they may open the road to a true insight into human nature and to a revision of the place man has assigned himself prior to his experience. Indeed, man experiencing pain will no longer consider himself as the measure of all things.[17]

Illness or the spectre of illness is a voice. It calls us from a complacent sense of being into an authentic sense of being. "The very fact that there is a quality of ought-ness about health, of ought-not-ness about illness and disease, suggests an ideal intention."[18]

This intentionality or directionality borne in the experience of disease is the first characteristic of the traditional view that illness is disruption. When the Tradition speaks of illness as a voice, it is initially an alarm or a call. At the very elementary level, pain can be a signal pointing to some deeper malady. It may also be the vivid reminder that healing, mending, and restoration are going on in the body and mind.

At a deeper level, we see that pain is the symbolic prefiguration of death. Disease is the forerunner of death. Death is not only the indicator of the misdirection in our lives, it is also the reminder of the possibility of redirection. In this sense, both sickness and mortality become a voice. Kierkegaard spoke of anxiety as rooted in our "sickness unto death." Primitive cultures, and perhaps the primitive sense in everyone, are aware of the fact that we are mortally ill. We will one day die. Disease reminds us of that fact. Surely the fear of and resistance to this signal is the volition that prompts the development of systems of biomedical knowledge as well as therapeutic attempts to overcome disease, debilitation, and death.

Karl Barth argues that it is our mortal illness, the fact that we are terminally ill, that makes possible our salvation.

> The liberation of man from the misery created by his sloth is a reality and therefore a living hope for all other men only in the crucified Jesus. To free us He took it to Himself. He made it His own misery. And as the bearer of it He could only die. It was only in His death that He could set this term to it; that He could make an end of it. A sickness which can terminate only with the death of the patient, from which he can be liberated only by death, is an incurable sickness, or one which can be cured only as it reaches its goal and end with the destruction of the sick person, thus coming up against a frontier which even it cannot pass. If Jesus is the patient for us, in our place, burdened with our sickness, it is obvious that we have to say of our sickness that as the misery to which the stupid and inhuman and dissipated and careworn man has fallen victim it is incurable—a fact which emerges with particular impressiveness in all the Old Testament passages to which we referred. Our first proposition is thus that it is a mortal sickness, i.e., that if we ourselves had to bear it, if Jesus had not carried it in our place, it could end only with our death and destruction.
>
> It does in fact end with our death to the extent that Jesus, burdened with our sickness, suffered our death. It is true that in His death, triumphing for us even as He suffered for us, He accomplished our new and healthy birth.[19]

The confrontation with impending death is a voice. The work of Elisabeth Kübler-Ross and the wide ranging literature on death and dying describe the way the voice of terminal illness is heard in the human being and how we transact subsequent experience in the light of that awareness. We attempt to not hear the voice, deamplify its power, muddle its signal. Finally, however, we focus the signal, listen to it with what can only be called anticipation. In the grand design of our creation we are structured to hear the message of God in the voice of illness. "God whispers to us in our pleasures," writes C. S. Lewis, "speaks in our conscience, but shouts in our pains. It is His megaphone to rouse a deaf world."[20]

Lewis has argued that the sense that human beings are mortally ill has receded in the modern mind. Through the myth of human invincibility and perfectability, we have obscured the signal. The "good man" myth, which we will consider in discussing the Experiment, has convinced us that since we are undeserving of death, we should set out boldly in the conquest of death. Lewis also claims that the broad movement of psychoanalysis has at its worst suggested that shame and guilt are not metaphysical. That is, they are not ethical mechanisms of the human spirit holding the possible and intended against the actual of our lives; rather, they are only repressions. These modern myths are so compelling that we have contorted illness into a voice that evokes fear and flight rather than challenge.

In the Christian tradition, illness is a voice for the purpose of our healing. The early theologians spoke of grace as the antidote to sin and sickness. Christ was called *pharmacos* and *iatros*; he is the Great Physician. Salvation is the rendering up to God of our disease; of receiving in grace powers of forgiveness and of mortification (literally, letting what is corruptible die so that the being might live); enduring with him the suffering for the sake of the joy that is set before us; being made whole, as in our death we are conformable to him.

HEALING AS CATHARSIS, SALVATION, AND RECONCILIATION

When John heard in prison about the deeds of the Christ, he sent word by his disciples and said to him, "Are you he who is come, or shall we look for another?" And Jesus answered them, "Go and tell

John what you hear and see: the blind receive their sight and the lame walk, and the poor have good news preached to them" (Matthew 11:2–5). And preach as you go, saying, "The kingdom of Heaven is at hand." Heal the sick, raise the dead, cleanse lepers, cast out demons. You received without pay, give without pay (Matthew 10:7–8).

He called the twelve together and gave them power and authority over all demons and to cure diseases, and he sent them out to preach the kingdom of God and to heal (Luke 9:1–2). When they heard it, they lifted their voices together to God and said, "Sovereign Lord, who didst make the heaven and the earth and the sea and everything in them. . . . And now, Lord, look upon their threats, and grant to thy servants to speak thy word with all boldness, while thou stretchest out thy hand to heal, and signs and wonders are performed through the name of thy holy servant Jesus" (Acts 4:24, 29–30).

In the preaching and ministry of the primitive New Testament community, the movement into life or the drama of salvation is seen as a progression from brokenness and alienation to being shocked into our senses by God's love come to us despite our rebellion. Then follows repentence, turning around, catharsis, and exorcism. Being made clean, we are healed, mended, made whole. Now well, we are restored to relatedness to self, to community, to God. Understood Christologically, pain becomes a signal of our human condition. Like an island lighthouse amid a stormy sea, it beckons us to awareness of what life is all about. The process of healing conveyed in the Christian drama is paralleled in other traditions. The element of confession and catharsis, for example, is present in most traditional forms of soul healing and psychiatry. "Laying bare" one's guilt has always had the effect of reducing anxiety and promoting healing. Even when personal prayer is regarded as monologue before some imaginary (placebo) deity, cathartic effect can be experienced.

A most interesting expression of this act in the drama is found in the confessions of the American Indians. Long before the missionary influence, Pueblo and Mexican tribes had the custom of making a least one full confession of sins during the lifetime. Especially in times of sickness were confessions invoked. For example, the Chol Maya

> were in the habit of confessing to their caciques [native chiefs] when sickness afflicted a member of the family, holding the belief that the sickness would end in death unless confession were made by son, father, or husband, etc. Should the whole community be suffering from plague or sickness, the confession of a serious sin would lead to the shooting of the sinner with bow and arrows.[21]

This aboriginal sense of seeing sin as the cause of sickness, and catharsis (either by confession or punishment of a scapegoat) as the prelude to healing, prefigures the universal sense of meaning that is conveyed in the Christian gospel. Here all pain is seen as part of the cosmic groaning, which, despite futility, yearns on in hope, knowing that the creation was "subjected to futility in hope" (Romans 8:18–20). This would seem to mean that the human anguish in the face of sickness and death is not absurd and ultimately futile but is a tempering experience that will eventually be transfigured into peace in the grand redemption now growing in creation.

As a summary of this first part of the book, let us look at one example of a metaphysic and of physic disease and health. John Wesley's *The Primitive Physick*[22] has had a great impact on personal health care and public health. The example will provide a window into the tradition, showing its wisdom and its weakness.

Several years ago, Robert Morison of Cornell University made a provocative statement at an annual meeting of The Hastings Institute. He suggested that the principal person and movement in the modern commitment to public health are

John Wesley and the Methodist Church. Having read Wesley's *Primitive Physick*, I found this rather surprising, because the manual is full of not only sound old wives' tales, but also many absurd curative concoctions. The asthmatic is urged to drink cold water before bed or take a cold bath. In fact, vasoconstriction has always brought relief to this malady. But for a "dry convulsive asthma," the reader is advised to "dry and powder a toad. Make it into small pills, and take one every hour till the convulsions cease."[23]

Morison claimed that, beyond the practical wisdom, Wesley introduced a fresh image of human life into Western culture: an image accenting cleanliness, purity, industry, and so forth. The human degradation rampant in the early stages of the industrial revolution and the factory movement was paralleled in most churches by a deprecation of the human body and a cynical disengagement from the social forces that demeaned human life. Wesley pleaded that people clean up, look up to Christ and be measured by his perfection, and transform the social instruments of business and industry into vessels that could abide Christ's appearing or at least be where people could walk "in his steps."

There is no doubt that we experienced a profound attitudinal change in the late eighteenth and early nineteenth centuries. Many forces converged, including the ability to clean streets, water supplies, and food sources; the first glimmerings of effective preventive and interventive medicine; the emergence of political reform movements; and the sensitization of the common conscience by writers like Charles Dickens and preachers like William Wilberforce. Perhaps the work of Wesley and his company was formative.

Primitive Physick was first published in 1747. Wesley himself regarded it as the best of his many publications.[24] The book went through twenty-three editions and was found in almost every English and American household, usually beside the Bible. Wesley lived in an age of brilliant medical insight and dismal medical care. The age of medical enlightenment was marked by men such as Loeuwenhoek, Harvey, Sydenham (whom Wesley extols in *Physick*), Lavoisier, Linnaeus, and Jenner. The emerging body of science had little effect, however, on the common people. As late as 1860, Oliver Wendell Holmes, the great American physician, could say: "If the whole *materia medica*, as now used, could be sunk to the bottom of the sea, it would be all the better for mankind—and all the worse for the fishes."[25]

Wesley sought to call the professions to be responsible servants to people. He sought as well to place tools for self-responsibility in the hands of all. He encouraged the family reading of the Bible, personal and family prayer, and devotion. He called on all to be diligent, disciplined, and joyous in the pursuit of well-being and godly conviviality, which were the earthly intimations of salvation.

He desired that common people have at their disposal the basic knowledge and therapies to treat illness. He wanted to give them "a plain and easy way of curing most diseases . . . to set down cheap, safe and easy medicines, easy to be known, easy to be procured, and easy to be applied by plain, unlettered men." When diseases persisted and the body did not proceed to heal itself with these assists, he advised "every man without delay to apply to a Physician that fears God."[26]

We note initially a strong trust in the common people. The virtues of medicine are rooted in this basic faith. Individuals are the best judges and final arbiters in decisions for their own good. The doctrine of informed consent and all the derivative statements of patients' rights are rooted in this central notion. It makes us realize how far we have strayed from this basic tenet when we see how we still debate the point, as if there were any earthly good that superceded the individual's own wish. By abandoning this precept, we have constructed a system based on passive reception of professional services and have lost the value of responsibility and self-care.

Wesley objected to the way in which the medical guild began appropriating to itself the secret body of knowledge and cures and set itself up as the dispenser of these mysteries.

> Physicians now began to be in admiration, as persons who were something more than human. And profit attended employ as well as honor; so that they had now two weighty reasons for their keeping the bulk of mankind at a distance, that they might not pry into the mysteries of the profession.[27]

The task of the profession should be to aid in preventing illness, maintaining health, and supporting the healing process for the sick. Patient and physician should together render themselves instrumental to the ministrations of the Great Physician. The noble physician is one who harkens back to traditional wisdom:

> Yet there have not been wanting from time to time, some lovers of mankind, who have endeavored, even contrary to their own interest, to reduce physick to its ancient standard, who have labored to explode it out of all the hypothesis and fine-spun theories, and to make it a plain intelligible thing, as it was in the beginning.[28]

In the background of Wesley's *Physick* is a theologically controlled world view which provides the backdrop for his pastoral counsels regarding health and disease. In the preface he writes:

> When man came first out of the hands of the Great Creator, clothed in body, as well as in soul, with immortality and incorruption, there was no place for physic, or the art of healing. As he knew no sin, so he knew no pain, no sickness, weakness, or bodily disorder. The habitation wherein the angelic mind, the Divine Particulae Aurae, abode, although originally formed of the dust of the earth, was liable to no decay. It had no seeds of corruption or dissolution within itself; and there was nothing without to injure it; heaven and earth, and all the host of them were mild, benign, and friendly to

human nature. The entire creation was at peace with man, so long as man was at peace with his Creator. So that well might the morning stars sing together, and all the sons of God shout for joy.

2. But since man rebelled against the Sovereign of heaven and earth, how entirely is the scene changed? The incorruptible frame hath put on corruption, the immortal hath put on mortality. The seeds of wickedness and pain, of sickness and death, are now lodged in our inmost substance; whence a thousand disorders continually spring, even without the aid of external violence. And how is the number of these increased by every thing round about us? The heavens, the earth, and all things contained therein, conspire to punish the rebels against their Creator. The sun and moon shed unwholesome influences from above: the earth exhales poisonous damps from beneath; the beasts of the field, the birds of the air, the fishes of the sea, are in a state of hostility; the air itself that surrounds us on every side, is replete with shafts of death; yea, the food we eat daily saps the foundation of that life which cannot be sustained without it. So has the Lord of All secured the execution of His decree—"Dust thou art, and unto dust shalt thou return."

3. But can nothing be found to lessen those inconveniences which cannot be wholly removed? To soften the evils of life, and prevent in part the sickness and pain to which we are continually exposed? Without question there may One grand preventative of pain and sickness of various kinds, seems intimated by the Grand Author of Nature in the very sentence that entails death upon us—"in the sweat of thy face shalt thou eat bread, till thou return to the ground." The power of exercise, both to preserve and restore health, is greater than can well be conceived; especially in those who add temperance thereto, who, if they do not confine themselves altogether to "Bread or the herb of the field," (which God does not require them to do) yet steadily observe both that kind and measure of food which experience shows to be most friendly to health and strength.

4. It is probable Physic, as well as Religion, was in the first ages chiefly traditional; every father delivering down to his sons what he had in like manner received, concerning the manner of healing

both outward hurts and the diseases incident to each climate, and the medicines which were of the greatest efficacy for the cure of each disorder.[29]

Note the elements: First there is a foundation theology. God gives the creation and creatures life and health. The disease in creation is of human making. Loren Eisely has noted that a great swirling whirlpool of destruction opens in the creation with the appearance of human beings. Yet God provides an antidote for sin. The perfections of Christ draw forth holiness from human life. This wholeness is found centrally in his work and prayer. This holiness is health. Consider one scenario of this traditional sense of meaning.

The Mullins family has moved to the Ohio frontier. A generation earlier the grandparents had emigrated from England and settled in New Jersey. Now the son and his young family have sought a new life on the rich farm lands of Ohio. Acreage has been cleared, and Mullins and his oldest son erect a simple log house. Weslyan revival has swept like fire across the frontier, and the Mullins family has been drawn into the local congregation. *The Primitive Physick* stands alongside the Bible on the fireplace mantle. The land is good and productive. God is praised for his bountiful provisions. Long days working the farm and evenings around the fire all contribute to a peaceful sense of contentment and well-being. Nature gives the seasons: springtime and harvest, planting and canning. Winter brings rest and school work, sewing and quilting, repairing tools for the next planting. Now mother is sick. A lump has grown in her stomach and she is losing weight. The doctor is summoned from a neighboring village. He can provide only some relief from pain. Some herbal drinks and remedies are tried from the *Physik*, but they provide only palliative comfort. Deep in the family's faith, they know that mother will die. She continues to weaken. One winter evening she calls the family together. She counsels and encourages the children and tenderly comforts her husband. Later that night she falls asleep, not to waken again. The pastor is summoned. A crude pine box is built by father and sons, and mother is buried on the hill behind the cabin. Friends and neighbors gather for the service. "The Lord gives, the Lord takes away," the preacher reads. "Blessed be the name of the Lord." Slowly, heads bowed, arm in arm, the family makes its way back down the hill. Hearts ache with loneliness, but underneath is found a trust that mother is at peace, and God is near to lead into tomorrow.

Note the characteristic elements. When sickness comes, only the body can cure. Disease must run its course. The physician and folk remedies can assist nature but only in very gentle ways. God is the companion of the sick. He brings his will out of the crisis. The family is drawn together. Close associations with the earth, with family, with neighbors are a strong support. Fate is accepted. Grief is accepted and expressed. Life goes on. All has its meaning in the divine purpose. These are the constituent elements of the Tradition. I will show in Chapters Three and Four how the Experiment, as part of mass-technological civilization, suspends many of these traditional elements, and how the Renovation seeks to recover them. Wesley writes: "The love of God is the sovereign remedy of all miseries. By the unspeakable joy and perfect calm serenity and tranquility it gives the mind, it becomes the most powerful of all the means of health and long life."[30]

This practical wisdom, together with its "Metaphysick," provides a glimpse of the Tradition. While the details may be found wanting or incorrect, the dispositions retain their validity. Human beings are travelers and sojourners in this world. They are afflicted. Yet even this flaw in existence can be understood in the overarching purpose of things and can be transformed into saving purpose, because God is Lord of all.

But people are not Tradition bound. The new taste of power and possibility led them to abandon some elements of the tradi-

tional culture with its theologies and rituals. With this new
freedom, conflicts, both intrapsychic and cultural, are set in
motion. Perhaps illness is not inescapable human destiny. Perhaps we need not suffer. Perhaps even death can be avoided.
An experimental mood is activated; a quest is set in motion. Yet
in the midst of the exhilaration, people wonder what they may
have lost. As Ivan Illich has written:

> All *traditional* cultures derive their hygienic function from this abil-
> ity to equip the individual with the means for making pain tolera-
> ble, sickness or impairment understandable, and the shadow of
> death meaningful. . . . Most healing is a *traditional* way of consoling,
> caring, and comforting people while they heal. . . . The ideology
> promoted by contemporary cosmopolitan medical enterprise runs
> counter to these functions.[31]

I have sketched the outline of a traditional sense of the
meaning of health and disease. In it, both disease and health
have a supernatural and metaphysical dimension. Disease is a
disruption, but a meaningful disruption in the light of the
traditional understanding of God and nature. Finally, healing
is a drama moving from brokenness to reconciliation. The Experiment questions these meanings and tests a novel interpretation of disease and health.

III

The Experiment

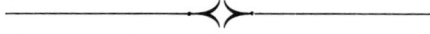

———————◇———————

THE DUKE: A man must come to terms with life as it is!
CERVANTES: I have lived nearly fifty years, and I have seen life
   as it is. Pain, misery, hungry . . . cruelty beyond belief. I
   have heard the singing from taverns and the moans from bun-
   dles of filth on the streets. I have been a soldier and seen my
   comrads fall in battle . . . or die more slowly under the lash in
   Africa. I have held them in my arms at the final moment.
   These were men who saw life as it is, yet they died despairing.
   No glory, no gallant last words . . . only their eyes filled with
   confusion, whimpering the question: "why?" I do not think
   they asked why they are dying, but why they have lived. When
   life itself seems lunatic, who knows where madness lives?
   Perhaps to be too practical is madness. To seek treasure where
   there is only trash. Too much sanity may be madness. And
   maddest of all, to see life as it is and not as it should be.

—*Man of La Mancha*[1]

"I must abide by medical tradition," said Robert Morse, the
attending neurologist in the Karen Anne Quinlan case. "I find
no medical precedent for withdrawing life-sustaining medical
procedures from a patient." Dr. Morse was quite certain that
the girl would never regain a "cognitive, functional existence."
Yet to grant the parents' request to spare "extraordinary
means" would violate current standards of medical practice.[2]

   "We just want to allow her to return to the arms of the Lord,"
said Mr. Quinlan from the stand. Their adopted daughter,

Karen Anne, had lain six months in coma. The mechanical respirator supported that vital function which rapidly diminishes when the device is withdrawn. The family believes in life after death and is devout in the Roman Catholic faith. "The earthly phase of her life has drawn to a close," said the family lawyer. "She should not be held back from enjoyment of a better, more perfect life."[3]

The two positions demonstrate the way the Tradition continues to coexist alongside the Experiment. Both moods claim divine sanctions. A theological impulse lies behind the mood we are calling the Experiment. God is seen as a partner in fighting evil, including disease, and a coworker in seeking life, and that in abundance. As human beings achieve new understandings and new powers, they begin to accent the themes of cocreativity with God in pursuing health as opposed to the more traditional accent on acceptance and resignation. The Experiment sets in motion an intense dialectic between assertiveness against disease and death and submission to the inevitable. Dietrich Bonhoeffer, who lived in profound tension between resistance and resignation, argued that modern people, blessed with science, must resist fate resolutely while learning to submit to it at the right time. The great scientist-philosopher Pierre Teilhard de Chardin writes:

> We must struggle against death with all our force, for it is our fundamental duty as living creatures. But when, by virtue of a state of things . . . death takes us, we must experience that paroxysm of faith in life that causes us to abandon ourselves to death as to a falling into a greater life.[4]

And resist, humanity has. Resistance is not uniquely modern; it has always been one side of mythic life. According to a Liberian legend, Sno-Nysoa, the Creator, sent his four sons to earth. After a time, he wanted them to return home to him, but they liked it on earth and wanted to remain. Earth, too, defied

Sno-Nysoa and tried to keep them. Thereupon God used his "secret power." One morning the eldest son could not wake up. God said to Earth: "I have simply called him home. I leave the body with you." Afterward, the same thing happened to the three remaining brothers—and all other human beings. Before Sno-Nysoa and Earth quarreled, death did not exist among human beings, but afterward there was sickness, suffering, and death.[5] This primal myth portrays the perpetual tension mortal beings feel with the Eternal Being.

The same tension was felt in the medical and parental opinions regarding Karen Anne Quinlan's fate. This is the crux of the theological difference between Tradition and Experiment. As history races forward, the argument between earth and the gods becomes intense. Life is found to be good and precious. We wish to cling to it. We cannot see life as the ancients did, a vale of tears. We find it difficult to concur with the Chorus in *Oedipus at Colonus*: "Never to have been born is best; and the next best, by far, to return thence, by the way speediest, where our beginnings are."[6] We cannot accept the contradiction of death, nor can we complacently abide death's prefiguration in disease. We decide to redirect the human quest into an Experiment of conquest.

From the perspective of nature alone, it can be argued that health is an idyllic and utopian state, while disease is the normal state. While I write this, the rubble is being removed following an earthquake in Guatemala. Tens of thousands are dead. Hundred of thousands are injured and sick from epidemic typhoid and other infections. A somber appraisal might see this catastrophe not as an aberration but as a collapse back to the tragic norm which is the bedrock character of our existence. The state of health, asepsis, epidemic control, managed preventive and interventive health care might be seen as a human contrivance, a construct holding back the basic malignant character of nature while providing us a temporary, suspended state of well-being. If disease and death are normative, then the Experiment becomes an expression of human ingenuity in keeping nature from reverting to its capricious self. In both the mythical and natural perspectives it is claimed that we are dealing with a human venture to offset the way uncontrolled supernature or nature would deal with human life.

The Tradition had to break down and undergo profound modifications. Indeed, the distortions in the Tradition lead to its rejection and to the initiation of the Experiment. Slowly but surely, a subtle change of attitude can be perceived in human history. We no longer resign ourselves before the apocalyptic spectre of the plagues. We set out to discover cause and cure. Catastrophic illness is not inevitable fate. Death becomes transfigured in Western art from a constant companion to a haunting visitor, then to an enemy which may prove vulnerable. Disease becomes a force to be dealt with and overcome.

Several subtle changes signal the transition from a traditional to an experimental understanding of the meaning of health and disease, symbolizing a new science of nature and a new theology. Before we delineate the characteristics of the Experiment, let us note a basic change in the world picture and a revision in understanding the healing act and role which together signal this movement toward a new experimental understanding of the meaning of health and disease.

In Hippocratic medicine we see the seeds of discontent with supernatural definitions of the etiology of disease. In the primitive understanding, the gods either directly intervened to punish human beings with the scourge of disease or abandoned them to the demons by withdrawing their protective care. In either case, sickness was sent as punishment and/or purification. Therefore, incantations accompanied medical therapies in all primitive traditions, serving either to invoke the deity or exorcise the malignant spirit.

Gradually a refinement occured in understanding the etiology of disease. In the air at the time of Hippocrates was the nature philosophy of ancient Greece which culminated in Aristotle. This tradition discerned various levels of causation in nature. In disease there is a material cause—the literal intermediary which brings about disease. The hemlock extract inflicts physical death. There is also what Aristotle would call formal causation. Life proceeds on the basis of an unfolding essence. It would be quite proper in this meaning to see disease as a change of life. It is not necessarily an invasion, a possession; it is the working out of certain physical and mental continuities. This latter sense eventually gave rise to the ontological, or what Aristotle might call the ontogenetic, view of disease. Disease is an entity which appears and disappears in human beings as certain formal predispositions and processes, growth and restoration, disintegration and decay continually interplay.

Glen Cunningham, an endocrinologist and internist at Baylor College of Medicine, intuits that we can best talk of the meaning of health and disease as spontaneous mutations, basic transformations in human life, which emerge because nature itself is creative. The emergences can be destructive or therapeutic. Nature continues to create anomalies or aberrations because its form is experimental; that is, nature is always innovating, always testing the novel.

Aristotle would also speak of a *causa finalis*, an ultimate (both spatially and temporally) purpose which is at work even in the disease process. God draws all life irresistably toward its purpose.

The Hippocratic physicians had this nuanced, Aristotelian mode of interpreting disease etiology. Demonic possession was too simple. There is certainly a demonic dimension in disease, but it is not sufficient cause. The organism must be ready to host disease. The environment must contribute the material cause. There are natural causes which deserve our rigorous examination. Riese makes the point with some overstatement: "Ever since Mediterranean civilization produced and adopted the Hippocratic system of medicine based on the action of natural phenomena, sacred elements have been banned from etiology."[7]

A careful study of the Hippocratic art, particularly the temple *Kurorts* where patients would sleep and convalesce, shows the deep sensitivity of Greek physicains to the spiritual and moral dimensions of healing. Yet the genius of the Hippocratic philosophy is its mythical-Pythagorean sense of the divine, which encouraged investigation of natural causes. Its theology of nature was one that encouraged knowledge; condemned ignorance, superstition, and dualistic demonism; and prompted investigative and therapeutic intervention. Nature will disclose its causes and the character of its processes if we observe carefully and reverently. The technical, manipulative inquiry where subject and object are split will probably not yield insight. The view of nature as enticing and revealing is a fundamental change from a primitive view which finds it foreboding and secretive.

The second change that signals the transition from Tradition to Experiment is an attitudinal one. We begin to look at those afflicted with disease neutrally, not judgmentally. In primitive tradition, the Down's syndrome child was "the holy idiot"; the epileptic was possessed with "the holy disease"; the young woman with schizophrenia was a witch. For the Hebrews, the hunchback or dwarf were ispo facto disqualified from the priesthood. In the Experiment the moral stigma attached to disease is diminished. Ther person who is sick is the victim of natural processes. Although he or she may have meaningfully participated in the causation and onset of the illness, the sufferer is not therefore deserving of either blame or praise.

From antiquity until the beginning of the present century, people with mental aberrations were seen as saints or devils, in touch with supernatural powers. An insane person was either held at a distance in awe or inflicted with the worst in torture and exorcism as an attempt to cleanse the tortured mind. Even Charles Bell's famous 1805 textbook on anatomy and neurology asserted that insanity was caused by sin. Slowly, both science and religion matured, rendering this superficial cause–effect relationship unacceptable. Today we cannot associate "sin" with madness as easily as earlier generations could. We do not readily designate masturbation as a disease nor as "drapetomania" (the slaves' compulsion to run away) necessarily a disorder.

Jung identifies the transition in this way:

> The ancient metaphysical explanation of Nature was discredited on account of its manifold errors. . . . In psychiatry during the first decades of the nineteenth century, the metaphysical exploration of nature ended in moralistic aetiological theories which explained neutral disease as a consequence of moral fault.[8]

I will argue in the final section of this book that we cannot completely diminish human moral responsibility and accountability in the realm of disease. Cancer is in some senses a disease phenomenon related to misuse of the environment and the technological life-style. We would not want to remove completely the moral factor from pulmonary diseases related to smoking, or from the range of diseases derivative of alcoholism. However, we did need to sever the simplistic causal ligature between disease and moral failure.

Out of this separation emerged a new and unfortunate polarization of the sciences and the humanities. Only now are we attempting to reintegrate the normative disciplines (those which probe what ought to be) with the descriptive disciplines (which describe what is). The role of scientist and humanist, of physician and priest, also separate. Rejecting the notion that spiritual impulses, psychic intentions, and moral qualities interplay in the onset, progress, and outcome of disease, the medical profession withdrew into a concept of healing which made the healer's role one of physical and technical manipulation. At the same time, the ministries of spiritual healing (cure of souls) withdrew to spiritualized notions of what happens in sickness and health. Christian Science represents the epitome of this reaction. Both divergencies depart from a sense of holiness and wholeness which can only flourish where a proper view of nature and the transcendent are held in conjunction.

In ancient cultures the roles of priest and healer were bound up in one person. In Judaism, as in most old oriental cultures, the moral guide and physician are one. In early Christianity the pastor and physical healer are often united. The apostles, as have been mentioned, were commanded and empowered to both proclaim the truth and heal the sick. In general, in the first millenium of the Christian era, the priest was physician. It is only in the early medieval world that the roles began to be differentiated. Medicine and the arts of physical diagnosis came to be suspect and condemned. Even though in the high middle ages, as in the Renaissance, the wise man who aspired to be a theologian had first to study science and medicine, the mood of distrust and condemnation came to prevail. Even as early as the sixth century, the Emperor Justinian I, convinced by church leaders, stifled the knowledge and art of medicine as spiritual action by closing the medical schools at Athens and Alexandria and withdrawing state support from both physicians and basic scientists. A series of papal edicts in the eleventh, twelfth, and thirteenth centuries forbade the study and practice of medicine and surgery by the clergy, thus placing the respected and noble arts in the hands of charlatans and barbers. Only in the monasteries did the unification of roles of pastor and physician, theologian and medical scientist endure. Healing was seen as the gift of God. Cassiodorus articulated the rule for a southern Italian monastery in the sixth century:

> I insist, brothers, that those who treat the health of the brethren . . .
> should fulfill their duties with exemplary piety. . . . Let them serve
> with sincere study to help those that are ailing, as becomes their
> knowledge of medicine, and let them look for their reward from
> Him who compensates temporal work by eternal wages. Learn
> therefore the nature of herbs, and study diligently the way to com-
> bine their various species for human health; but do not place your
> entire hope on herbs, nor seek to restore health only by human
> counsels. Since medicine has been created by God and since it is He
> who gives back health or restores life, turn to Him.[9]

Unfortunately, the rigor of this intellectual synthesis and the unification of roles of spiritual and physical healing did not prevail. It remains for the now-appearing Renovation to begin the new synthesis.

As I describe the Experiment, the reader should keep in mind that the Tradition in its folk aspect and its religious di-mension still lives in the human community just beneath the surface of the dominant scientific mentality. Some patients at the cancer center where I work have been known to supple-ment Prednisone and L. Asparaginase with their own con-coctions of pulverized rattlesnake when being treated for leukemia. At present, the traditions of folk medicine, soul heal-ing, psychiatry, psychoanalysis, and pastoral counseling consti-tute parallel healing activities and concurrent notions of the meaning of illness and disease. This persistent presence of the Tradition even in the bastions of scientific medicine shows that we still need to assimilate the values of the Tradition into our modern scientific consciousness.

The term *Experiment* is used deliberately to capture the significance of an era. To be arbitrary, we might say the Experiment begins with Descartes' nocturnal vision of universal mechanics in 1619 and ends in 1947 with the Nuremberg trials, the final despiritualization and demoralization of medicine. The glory and tragedy of medical experimentation is found during this period.

Viewing the human body as machine has enabled medical science to understand systems, physical dynamics, neurological electrics, and so forth. This has yielded technological skills such as monitoring fluids and electrolytes; supporting, even replacing, physical functions; artificial respiration; renal dialysis; anesthesia; antibiotic therapy; and the wide range of chemotherapies. Indeed, the entire modern armamentarium used to stabilize and sustain the human body in traumatic crisis was born in the empirical genius of the Experiment.

Similarly, the dehumanizations to which we have fallen subject are derivative of this novel experiential handling of the human organism in terms of knowledge and technique. The medical investigations undertaken by the Third Reich physicians included experiments testing human response to high altitude, freezing, malaria, sulfanilamide, jaundice, and spotted fever. These experiments often ended in death for the experimental subjects as well as sterilization, euthanasia, and execution of various deformed or "abnormal" persons. The final solution to ensure racial health and racial purity was to exterminate the "valueless lives" (*Lebensunwerten Lebens*).

One example will show the mood that characterizes the Experiment. The symbolic meaning of "laying on hands" changes with this new mentality. The change occurred in Greek medicine.

While the magic physician turned in diagnosis through divinations to regions far away from the patient himself, namely the dwelling places of supernatural forces, the Greek physician made through palpation the patient himself the most direct and intimate source of knowledge. Palpation symbolizes the physician's successful effort to bring the patient into the orbit of his own power and to detach him definitely from supernatural forces.[10]

Here we see conjoined the brilliance and the tragedy of the Experiment. The strength of the new approach is that imaginary spiritual energies projected on some extraneous source of divination, forces alien and alienating, are repudiated. The person—touched in palpation, physical exam, and the laying on of hands—is affirmed. In a sense, the doctor is saying to the patient: "No outside force will harm you; you are in my hands. Place yourself in my trust—under my control—and all will go well." The tragedy of this facet of the Experiment is that it seeks to ignore the relatedness of the living God, the holy healing Spirit, in the transactions of our personal life. Dürer's praying hands and the faith healers' instrumental hands are contorted into manipulative hands. Like the Hebrews at the gate of the promised land, we are tempted to say, "My strength and the power of my hands have gotten me this wealth" (Deuteronomy 8). Unless there is no God, is it not wiser to affirm the cooperation of our hands with his, our works and his? The Renovation physician, laying on hands, can see touch both as control and instrumentality to divine healing.

MAN AS MASTER

I now turn to an analysis of the experimental sense of human nature, the meaning of disease and health, and the nature of healing. Although one of the insights of the Experiment is to question human distinctiveness from nature and affirm the fact that human beings rise within nature (Aristarchus through Darwin), the Experiment stresses man as master, not as microcosm. At the eve of the First World War, William Osler stated somewhat ecstatically that man was now master on the earth.

> To have lived through an epoch, matched only by two in the story of the race, to have shared in its long struggle, to have witnessed its final victory (and in my own case, to be left I trust with wit enough to realize its significance—to have done this has been a wonderful privilege. To have outgrown age-old theories of man and nature, to have seen west separated from east in the tangled skein of human thought, to have lived in a world re-making —these are among the thrills and triumphs of the Victorian of my generation. To a childhood and youth came echoes of the controversy that Aristarchus began, Copernicus continued and Darwin ended, that put the microcosm in line with the macrocosm, and for the golden age of Eden substituted the tellus dura of Lucretius. Think of the Cimmerian darkness out of which our generation has, at any rate, blazed a path! . . . An age of force followed the final subjugation of nature. The dynamo replaced the steam engine, radiant energy revealed the hidden secrets of matter, to the conquest of the earth was added the control of the air and the mastery of the deep. Nor was it only an age of force. Never before had man done so much for his brother. The victory over the powers of nature meant also glorious victories of peace, pestilences were checked, the cry of the poor became articulate, and to help the life of the submerged half became the sacred duty of the other. How full we were of the pride of life! In 1910 at Edinburgh I ended an address on "Man's Redemption of Man" with the well-known lines of Shelley beginning "Happiness and Science dawn though late upon the earth."[11]

Scholars offer varying interpretations of the historical and intellectual developments that brought about this change in people's concept of their role in nature. Social analysts see a direct correlation with the collapse of the religious world view. David Mechanic notes, however, that "throughout much of the world today people still seek help from their ills from diviners, witch doctors, and other healers—often at the same time they use the facilities of modern medicine." This somewhat contradictory behavior is particularly true in cultures that are in the transition from traditional to modern mentality. The change occurs, however, because of a "growing diminution of the authority of religious conceptions of bodily functions and a growing dependence on a medical conception of physical experience." Even people who retain a strong religious world view and life-style abandon spiritual and moral interpretations of health and illness. "One of the most impressive characteristics of modern technological notions is the extent to which life conceptions, previously within the province of morals and religion, have been removed to the technical sphere."[12] This analysis suggests not so much that man is master but that he is no longer mastered. No forces extraneous to nature are thought to affect him. The Experiment sees life in an autonomous, not heteronomous, way.

Another perspective, popular in scientific circles, would say that human beings gain a sense of mastery as they come to understand natural phenomena. The emergence of the modern scientific intellect, building on the work of Occam, Cusanus, Galileo, and Newton, down to Darwin and the modern scholars of physics and natural science, is convinced that better knowledge of causes and effects, of processes and patterns has rendered humanity less vulnerable to the caprice of nature and more its master.

I have been intrigued in recent years by yet another interpretation. It may be helpful to look at the transformations in the mythology of Western culture in forming the notion that man is master over nature. Some have claimed that there exists even in the Hebrew idea of man as lord in nature (Genesis 1:28) the idea of domination. Closer examination shows that the Hebrew theme of human dominion in the creation is much more an affirmation of the fact that we are creatures—caretakers and stewards—rather than masters.

Alfred North Whitehead and others have built upon this theological root an interpretation of why the West has become a scientific and technological civilization. More convincing is the idea that the Western sense of mastery over nature is derivative of a mythology quite alien to Judeo-Christianity. Greece, though fundamentally a religious civilization, held the myth that humans are partners with the gods in the transactions of nature and history, fellow warriors against the fiends, demons, and apocalyptic horsemen that thunder through history. Even in the Greek pantheon, the gods become capricious, subject to foibles. As the sense of wonder, mystery, and transcendence diminishes, people come to see the gods weaker and themselves stronger. The primal Greek myth of *götterdammerung* is transmuted into the modern symbol of the twilight of the gods. The gods observe that humanity is come of age, that its powers over nature are like their own. Humans perceive that they themselves are possessed with godlike prehension and power. The modern mood, signified by Nietzsche, Wagner, and Freud, affirms the power and mastery of humanity and the weakness and irrelevance, if not absence, of the gods. We see ourselves as the giver and taker of life, the modern Prometheus who harnesses energy to his will. All the while, in the glow of conquest and accomplishment we feel ambivalent, perhaps even ashamed for usurping the divine prerogatives. We sense a certain force of judgment, retribution, and contradiction to our actions. Nemesis breathes on our pretensions. Eric Kahler's great study of the German character portrays this ambivalence.

> In the conquering Germanic chieftains, [the] ambivalent situation was reflected in a deeply ambivalent state of mind. Confronted with the intangible power and prestige of Rome, they vacillated between physical force and respectful humility. Victorious Germanic chieftains who took possession of Roman territories were suddenly paralyzed by some mysterious fear or shame or repentence. They felt the need to submit to what they had subjugated.[13]

Whatever the precipitating factors, an unprecedented sense of mastery controls the human self-estimate in the Experiment. The period and the mood contain several elements. Let us note the intellectual and attitudinal significance of this outlook.

Scientific materialism and physicalistic reductionism become intellectual criteria to understand and explain what is going on in nature. This becomes a pivotal feature of the Experiment. Beginning with Descartes, a way of approaching nature develops wherein matter is seen in mathematical and mechanical terms. Meanwhile, the phenomena of thought and value are said to belong to another realm. While scientists of the Experiment do not deny the transcendent, and indeed may be religious, they generally claim that the spiritual cannot be empirically known and therfore is not relevant for a working picture of reality.

Human beings are an intersection of mind and matter, of idea and thing, of subject and object, of the nomenal and phenomenal zones of reality. As such, they are master, arbiter, planner, interpreter of nature. Out of this world view emerges a style of encountering and handling nature, treating it objectively, fragmenting it into understandable parts, and managing it manipulatively. In this view, human nature itself is objectified and comes to be thought of as manipulable.

Analysis of the intellectual meaning of this revolution of thought is well developed.[14] For our purpose we should note that human beings come to be seen as mathematically discernible creatures. That is, our systems and the processes of life can be quantified, calculated, predicted, modeled, and programed. Our vital functions—blood flow; cellular development; heart, lung, kidney and other organ action; even brain functions—can be understood in terms of biophysics and mathematics and can be treated mechanically. The human body as a machine becomes the prevalent model of experimental medicine.

The shift in attitude that accompanies this shift in conceptualization is equally critical in understanding the Experiment.

No longer is an attitude of acceptance and resignation before nature acceptable. Submission is transformed into domination. Gotthard Booth, a physician who has written extensively on issues at the interface of theology and medicine, claims that down through the ages people most often lived in peaceful symbiosis with bacteria. Only when the body became vulnerable from malnutrition, emotional stress, old age, and so on, did germs get the upper hand. Today, at least in the scientific West, we see the ascendency of neoplastic diseases over infectious diseases. The change is not simply the result of medical progress, Booth argues; it is a reflection of a basic attitudinal shift from passivity to control.

> The connection between technological progress and the changing balance of infectious and cancerous diseases is not simply an unfortunate by-product of certain scientific inadequacies of medicine. The root of both developments is found in the emergence of a new personality type. The so-called conquest of nature is not the result of intellectual advance, but of a different motivation in the use of the intellect.[15]

Although the etiology of cancer is much more complex than Booth suggests, it may be true that some broad psychosomatic factors are involved with this disease, just as they are involved in generalized obsessive-compulsive neurosis and stress-induced disease. Many illnesses in the modern world are symptoms of a posture toward nature which seeks to dominate and control. Others are induced perhaps by passivity and "giving up." Either approach finds expression in both personal psychic structure and cultural style.

The shift in attitude toward disease from acceptance to control was accompanied by the basic intellectual change from metaphysical and teleological to mechanistic world views. We began at this point to see people differently: as machines, systems of parts and processes which could be separated, isolated, and manipulated. Institutions of care and educational programs for physicians and nurses both changed to accomodate this conceptual shift. We are master. We now organize our scientific quest around the assumption that we can know and control. This basic estimate of human power now begins to modify our sense of the meaning of disease.

DISEASE AS DISRUPTION

Disease can no longer be easily rationalized within some grand scheme of meaning. It certainly cannot be written off as the working of some obscure supernatural forces. The new mode of understanding has no need for metaphysical factors. God has nothing to do with sickness and health. Loss accompanies the gain, since in ignoring these referential aspects of sickness, both healer and patient are robbed of contexts of meaning.

Although it is true that patient and physician in some ways begin to interpret the particular treatments of medicine as objective interventions, spiritually and morally neutral, the deeper meaning in the experiences of healing and suffering continues. In demythologizing health and disease, the Experiment both gains as it abandons fallacious elements in the Tradition and loses as it fails to hold onto elements of enduring value.

Diseases come to be seen as great disruptions in the fabric of nature. Illich argues that the nineteenth century began to interpret diseases as entities having formidable power and personality in and of themselves.

> We have seen death turn from God's call into a "natural" event and later into a "force of nature"; in a further mutation it is now turned into an "untimely" event unless coming to those who were both healthy and old. Now it had become the outcome of specific disease certified by the doctor.

Death has paled into a metaphorical figure, and killer diseases have taken his place. The general force of nature that had been celebrated as "death" turned into a host of specific causations of clinical demise. Many "deaths" now roam the world. A number of book plates from private libraries of late nineteenth century physicians show the doctor battling with personified diseases at the bedside of his patient. The hope of doctors to control the outcome of specific diseases gave rise to the myth that they had power over death.[16]

A radically new sense of meaning is brought to disease and health in the Experiment. Although the Tradition sees disease as tragic, it is still a part of nature; it is to be borne courageously; it can be purposive in the grand scheme of things. Now we see that a different sense of disease and health has emerged. What is the working assumption of the nature of physical and mental disease that we find in the Experiment?

Before we deal with this question, it must be noted that the fundamental assumption of the early modern mind is that no purpose can be discerned in physical process. This idea has its roots in Newtonian physics, where nature is conceived as a vast perpetual motion apparatus, the great machine. In the words of Niels Bohr, "In this so-called classical mechanics all reference to purpose is eliminated, since the course of events is described as automatic consequence of given initial conditions."[17] The new world view also has roots in Cartesian philosophy, where nature had been made "a machine and nothing but a machine; purposes and spiritual significance had alike been banished."[18] Eventually, the wheels set in motion by Descartes destroy even that which he sought to protect. Human thought and value, *res cognitans*, the realm of thought, is brought within the "empirical reach," and all human behavior comes to be mechanistically understood within the model of physicalistic reductionism. Life scientists come to feel "that physiological and mental processes must ultimately be reducible to mechanical motions of atoms and corpuscles, and that, accordingly, all the imperfection of causal explanations which we observe can only be provisional."[19] We may not yet know the physio-chemical process involved when we experience anger or ecstasy, but one day we will. Then we will have "mood rings" that will record many parameters of the body's response to stress, and we will be able to make the appropriate corrections.

The significance of this basic characteristic of scientific inquiry is just beginning to be seen as the root of our value crisis today. As we look at the human person as well as at the ecosphere, we realize the necessity and yet the distortion of looking reductionistically at parts isolated from the whole. The biologist Barry Commoner locates in environmental science the same flaw that distorts human science and technology.

> There is, indeed, a specific fault in our system of science, and in the resultant understanding of the natural world which, I believe, helps to explain the ecological failure of technology. This fault is reductionism, the view that effective understanding of a complex system can be achieved by investigating the properties of its isolated parts. The reductionist methodology, which is so characteristic of much of modern research, is not an effective means of analyzing the vast natural systems that are threatened by degreadation.[20]

This fundamental view of the nature of physical process comes to control the Experiment's sense of what disease and health are. All disease is simply meaningless perturbation of physical process. Some diseases are maladaptations or over-adaptations in the evolutionary process. Diabetes, sickle-cell disease, Tay-Sachs disease, perhaps Down's syndrome, and even cancer are distorted physical processes that *are* rooted in the long genetic human evolution. The origin of the mutation may have originally been for protection; the sickle-cell and Tay-Sachs traits are thought to have originally been protective mutations against malaria and tuberculosis. Air- and water-borne infections disturb the normal process of the cells and introduce pathogenic process. The ideopathic diseases, those in which organs, tissues, vessels, and so forth break down, are the results of various loads and pathologies in those cells. Cancer becomes a fundamentally cellular disturbance. Something begins to happen which is very like the creation of life itself. In mental illness certain neurochemical or neuroelectrical patterns are disturbed.

The new sense of the nature of disease, when considered in this composite fashion, is that all disease is aberration, anomaly, disturbance. Basic physical process has been disrupted. It can be corrected, if not now, later. All of the human processes—endocrinal, metabolic, neurological—are at the deepest level atomic transactions, physiochemical processes which can be understood and modified. Aging itself—a phenomenon of cellular loads triggered by genetic factors—is a physical process amenable to alteration.

The central character of the Experiment is shaped when this scientific notion of physicalistic reductionism is joined to the Nordic myth of conquest. The Nordic myth takes root in Northern Europe, Scandinavia, Scotland, and Germany, those cultures where the industrial revolution and later the emergence of high technological civilization began. Arianism, we will recall, is the form of Christianity that was repudiated in southern Europe and Africa but gained a foothold in the North. The cardinal tenet of Arianism is the humanity of Jesus, the divinity of human beings. A related tendency, Pelegianism, deemphasizes human sin. This mentality, common to the Goths, Franks, and Burgundians, persisted despite the normalizing of Athanasian, trinitarian Roman Christianity. It shaped the theology of the Northern European Reformation. Since the Reformation the repeated appearance of Arminianism in Northern Europe, a view which emphasized the human factor in salvation, is an eruption of this older theological strain. The legacy of the myth is that there is no transcendent power worth worrying about. We are Lord in the earth. At least in this world, God's work is our own (J. F. Kennedy), or in this world we must be responsible not *to* but *for* God (Dag Hammarskjold).

In his brilliant portrayal of *The Ascent of Man*, Jacob Bronowski ventures an opinion as to why the early flourishing of science occurred in Italy, but it remained for Northern Europe to take the revolution to its fruition. Bronowski finds the critical event to be the trial of Galileo by the Inquisition. In my interpretation, it is not only the force of the Church but the fact that both the common and the great believed in the Church. We sense in Galileo the mood that perhaps, indeed, he *is* wrong. The recantation is not merely a coerced confession; he is genuinely remorseful.

In the North, the trial of Luther, for example, reveals a completely different world view, a greater willingness to challenge authority, a larger spirit of inquisitiveness and iconoclasm. The apotheosis of man and the glorification of the physician are the legacies of this cultural myth. Science and technology in the modern spirit find their origins in Germany, Poland, Scandanavia, Scotland, and England, becoming the national soil for the industrial revolution and the derivative culture of high technology.

Modern medicine in this spirit sees itself engaged in a conquest of disease. We have proclaimed a war on cancer and blood vessel disease. In Pakistan and East Africa we are now tracking down the last lingerings of smallpox in the world. The eradication in the Western world of the once devastating childhood diseases is but a symbol of the larger conquest of infectious disease. The Nordic warrior armed with the *Merck Manual* and the *Physician's Desk Reference* is now ready to attack those remaining enemies: cancer and mental illness and the lingering ideopathic diseases. We are not sure where to attack, because our books and our strategy, our knowledge and intervention technology, are still in the formative stage. We are also unsure where to initiate the attack because we fear that the enemy may retreat and advance around the flank and attack at another point. The forced mutations in the microbiological world may one day gain the upper hand. Some future flu virus strain may defy the vaccine. The cure may be worse than the disease. The substituted disease of treatment may be worse than the natural disease.

Yet the modern Faust remains poised for the battle, not sure—and perhaps not caring—whether his soul be damned or saved. Underlying both his knowledge and his attitude is aggression. Disease is a disruption to be smoothed out and explained, a disturbance to be calmed, an anomaly to be corrected, a voice to be silenced. The question that remains is whether we can survive this dream or whether it will become a nightmare.

Several writers have pointed to the unreality, fantasy, and perhaps even danger in the view that biomedical warriors must crusade against and eradicate disease from the human realm. Peter Sedgwick has suggested that our designation of some natural phenomena as disease is quite arbitrary and value laden. Our concepts of disease are in one sense only "social conventions."

> All departments of nature below the level of mankind are exempt both from disease and from treatment. The blight that strikes at corn or at potatoes is a human invention, for if man wished to cultivate parasites rather than potatoes (or corn) there would be no "blight" but simply the necessary foddering of the parasite-crop. Animals do not have diseases either, prior to the presence of man in a meaningful relation with them. . . . Outside the significances that man voluntarily attaches to certain conditions, there are no illnesses or diseases in nature. . . . Out of his anthropocentric self-interest, man has chosen to consider as "illnesses" or "diseases" those natural circumstances which precipitate the death (or the failure to function according to certain values) of a limited number of biological species: man himself, his pets and other cherished livestock, and the plant-varieties he cultivates for gain or pleasure. . . . Children

and cattle may fall ill, have diseases, and seem as sick, but who has ever imagined that spiders or lizards can be sick or diseased? . . . The medical enterprise is from its inception value-loaded; it is not simply an applied biology, but a biology applied in accordance with the dictates of social interest.[21]

In contrast to Sedgwick, the Experiment has focused its attention on the physical basis, the ontological reality of disease. In an historical essay, Chester Burns shows the way in which this concept developed.[22] Initially, there was the Hippocratic view that diseases are natural phenomena. Then came the ontological view in which diseases were seen to be discrete entities with natural histories. The germ theory in the nineteenth century emphasized the fact that diseases were entities. Pathologists in the late nineteenth and early twentieth centiries explained disease in terms of anatomical, physiological, and pathological characteristics. This stream of thought would not admit that disease classification was a value. It was observable fact.

In an even more telling argument, Illich posits that diseases are indeed natural phenomena, that our repsonses to these processes are, of course, value laden, but the tone of our conquering mood, knowledge-based, mythically empowered, technologically implemented, is sadly misguided. Our medical interventions have not significantly altered the ebb and flow of disease patterns in the history of nature. Indeed, if the burden of disease and mortality are constant in nature and human experience, we may only be rearranging the topography of the disrupted landscape, making it more precarious and more dangerous to the human life experience. Medical progress, in making it more difficult for nature to claim our lives in death, may be ensuring that we suffer in more intense and excruciating ways.

The infections that prevailed at the outset of the industrial age illustrate how medicine came by its reputation. Tuberculosis, for instance, reached a peak over two generations. In New York in 1812, the death rate was estimated to be higher than 700 per 10,000; by 1882, when Koch first isolated and cultured the bacillus, it had already declined to 370 per 10,000. The rate was down to 180 when the first sanatorium was opened in 1910, even though "consumption" still held second place in the mortality tables. After World War II, but before antibiotics became routine, it had slipped into eleventh place with a rate of 48. Cholera, dysentery, and typhoid similarly peaked and dwindled outside the physician's control. By the time their etiology was understood and their therapy had become specific, these diseases had lost much of their virulence and hence their social importance. The combined death rate from scarlet fever, diphtheria, whooping cough, and measles among children up to fifteen shows that nearly 90 percent of the total decline in mortality between 1860 and 1965 had occurred before the introduction of antibiotics and widespread immunization. In part this recession may be attributed to improved housing and to a decrease in the virulence of micro-organisms, but by far the most important factor was a higher host-resistance due to better nutrition. In poor countries today, diarrhea and upper-respiratory-tract infections occur more frequently, last longer, and lead to higher mortality where nutrition is poor, no matter how much or how little medical care is available. In England, by the middle of the nineteenth century, infectious epidemics had been replaced by major malnutrition syndromes, such as rickets and pellagra. These in turn peaked and vanished to be replaced by the diseases of early childhood and, somewhat later, by an increase in duodenal ulcers in young men. When these declined, the modern epidemics took over: coronary heart disease, emphysema, bronchitis, obesity, hypertension, cancer (especially of the lungs), arthritis, diabetes, and so-called mental disorders. Despite intensive research, we have no complete explanation for the genesis of these changes. But two things are certain: the professional practice of physicians cannot be credited with the elimination of old forms of mortality or morbidity, nor should it be blamed for the increased expectancy of life spent in suffering from the new diseases.[23]

Leon Kass, I assume, would agree with Illich in recognizing disease as physical phenomena that by nature are deleterious. Finding offense in disease is not simply a human evaluative construct. Illness is an experience that draws out moral response from us. Yet we cannot intensify our moral abhorrence and correlative corrective hope into unrealistic expectations and efforts in the pursuit of some abstract "ideal" of health. The end achieved might be very dangerous to our health.

Kass would argue that health, illness, and unhealth are indeed real. They exist "even if not discovered and attributed."[24] The question is how we morally perceive these values and what we do on the basis of that evaluation. Perhaps life should be lived courageously in the presence of disruption and flaw; we should not resign ourselves to disease where its remedy is in the service of wholeness and well-being but temper our conquering spirit in the service of more human values. Disease and finitude are to be courageously experienced, not defied or obliterated in our passion for invincibility.

An important related clinical perspective is brought to bear on the Experiment's understanding of disease in Mark Zborowski's excellent study, *People in Pain*. The survey is made of several ethnic groups to see what variations occur in response to disease and pain in New York hospitals. The thesis is that Irish, Italian, and Jewish attitudes towards pain (expressive, communal, etc.) gradually modulate in the second and third generations to become more like the "old American" attitude which represses the desire to scream and moan and sees pain as something to be excised at any cost!

The old American attitude (Scots-English or German ancestry) sees the body as a mechanism. Pain has only a biological function. When hospitalized, the sufferer focuses on techniques, facilities, food, and so forth, and is inclined towards surgical excision of whatever it is that hurts. Zborowski reflects on this attitude, which shows our American sense of the character of sickness as disruption or eruption to be excised.

> Health is seen as the most important asset in the individual's pursuit of his life goals and in his constant struggle for a better job, for more financial security, and for happiness in the family circle. Health is a primary condition for employment, for a normal marriage and for successful relations with people. If health is poor or impaired, the individual is strongly handicapped in his social and economic activities. It places him in a subordinate and disadvantaged position in relation to the competitive processes of society. Furthermore, he becomes an emotional and financial burden to his community and his family, and he may be avoided or sometimes even isolated from healthy people by the walls of hospitals and sanitariums. Illness deprives the individual of his most valued prerogatives: independence and self-reliance. Illness is often equated and identified with old age, that is, the most undesirable period of human life, when "the body deteriorates, when something keeps one in bed, and makes me a burden for someone for a long time."[25]

In summary, the experimental mood in our culture and epoch in our history introduces a new value regarding the meaning of disease. The main impact of this new sense is that disease is value free; it has no meaning; it is absurd, morally and spiritually neutral. The view emerges first as a diverging trend within the dominant religious-moral tradition of Hebrew, Hippocratic, and Arabic medicine. In Renaissance and modern medical thought, the view becomes stronger, eventually becoming normative in the Experiment. Aarne Siirala summarizes:

> When the main course of Western medicine began to take shape in the midst of this cultural tradition, however, there occurred in the understanding of illness a radical departure from the mythological tradition. The development began in Greek culture, where students of nature (physiologoi) gathered the material for theories of the structure of nature (physis). It was on this basis that the first

"natural" explanations of the character of illness were built. Corpus Hippocraticum gathered and canonized views which described illness as a phenomenon of nature. Thus illness was regarded in the Hippocratic tradition as a disturbance of the equilibrium which rules in nature. In the treatment of illness the aim was to find the natural causes of the disturbance and to restore the proper balance. The task of the physician was to be "the servant of nature." He was required to understand the structure of nature and to seek immediate causes of illness in the human body, more remote causes in universal nature. The goal of medical care was seen to be the healing or elimination of the sick "elements" of the human organism, and this was to be based on a knowledge of the structure of nature, a knowledge reached through empirical research. All forms in which illness appeared, both physical and psychic, were to be studied as symptoms of disturbances in the human organism.[26]

HEALING AS MANIPULATION

Healing in the Experiment is achieved when disturbance is removed and equilibrium is restored. Therapeutics are, for the most part, manipulative. In inherited disorders, for example, attempt is made to offset the deleterious effect of the sickness. Cure is impossible. The basic genetic structure, at least at this time, cannot be modified. The child with PKU disease is prescribed a diet low in phenylalanine and the devastating effects of mental retardation are avoided. Recombinant DNA modification may one day effect an even more basic control. The diabetic treated with insulin is both protected from the terror of acute episodes and coma and allowed to live to bear children and experience the devastations of end-stage diabetes.

In the field of genetic disease, there is a race occurring between two competing biophilosophies. One view argues that we should perfect our manipulative and corrective therapeutics and technologies and learn how to make life bearable for people even with profound inherited disease. Some argue that we will soon have adequate knowledge and corrective treatment to allow children to survive with Tay-Sachs disease. The same argument is made regarding Duschene's muscular dystrophy and cystic fibrosis. A few scientists even argue that the physical morbidity introduced by the trisomy anomaly in Down's syndrome may be prevented.

The other view argues that our manipulative therapeutics should concentrate on using prenatal diagnosis, sharpening our tools of reading markers on the genes and chromosomes, and aborting those children who carry these inherited defects. We will thus, it is argued, give other children who may not bear these deficiencies the opportunity to be born. Although we may be inclined toward one option or the other, it should be noted that both approaches rest on the impulse to control and not accept what is; and both advocate manipulations as the therapeutic response.

Genetic disease is transmissable disease. Unlike other varieties of communicable disease, it is passed on with mathematical predictability via vertical, as opposed to horizontal, transmission. What preventive and therepeutic goals should we pursue in the law and in science policy? Burying our heads in the sand will no longer do. We cannot possess knowledge and feign ignorance and passive inaction. This terrible cost of our freedom is understood by the Experiment.

In the range of sicknesses that affect us during the course of our lives, the Experiment also sees healing as manipulation and management. If we are afflicted with viral, bacterial, or fungal infections, antibiotic agents are introduced to assist the body's resistance. If lesions appear in the organs of the body, surgery is called on to excise, reroute vessels, or otherwise correct the flaw. In psychological disorder, various modes of chemotherapy and psychotherapy are undertaken. Most often the objective is to reclaim the capacity to function in a meaningful way.

At the gerontological end of the spectrum, the essence of the medical effort is manipulation to enable people to continue functional existence despite the slow onset of degenerative processes and acute traumas. Blood pressure is managed; the injury and debilitation of stroke is diminished by rehabilitation therapy; a failing heart and occluded vessels are managed if not with surgery then with life-style, exercise, and diet controls. Malignant growths are either surgically removed or controlled with chemical, immunological, or radiation therapy. In the dying process, fluids, electrolytes, and metabolites are medically controlled; infections are treated with antibiotics. Life supports are introduced to assist failing functions.

We come to the hospital for treatment. Each disease entity has a treatment of choice. Science has yielded a preferred treatment. It is very difficult to raise the issue of *no* treatment or a variety of treatment options. To request medical care is to submit to medical treatments. Medicine in the Experiment is schooled to do something—to control, to modify, to manipulate. This becomes its glory and its potential tragedy.

When the forces of scientific reductionism, medical specialization with a focus on diseases and body parts, and manipulative therapeutics combine, then depersonalization, the very antithesis of healing, can ensue. Tolstoy addressed this issue in *The Death of Ivan Illyich*.

The doctor said: this-and-that indicates that this-and-that is wrong with you, but if an analysis of this-and-that does not confirm our diagnosis, we must suspect you of having this-and-that, then . . . and so on. There was only one question Ivan Illyich wanted answered: was his condition dangerous or not? But the doctor ignored that question as irrelevant. From the doctor's point of view, such a question was unworthy of consideration. One had only to weigh possibilities: floating kidneys, chronic catarrh, or an ailment of the caecum. There was no question of the life of Ivan Illyich— nothing but a contest between floating kidneys and the caecum. In the presence of Ivan Illyich the doctor gave a brilliant solution to the problem in favor of the caecum, with the reservation that the analysis of his water might supply new information necessitating a reconsideration of the case.[27]

The meaning we bring to death has transmuted under the impact of the Experiment. As I write these words, a tall crane constructing a twelve-story hospital fifty feet from my office has accidentally snared a platform and dropped a worker twelve stories to his death. An accident; who is to blame? The crane operator is delirious and confused in his anguish. Capricious fate; why this forty-five year old man with small children? Why him? Now? No one right now can rationalize this as a timely death. His time had come. God was ready for him. No! Blind absurdity! Our sense of death as an aspect of patterned meaning has receded with respect to both unexpected and expected deaths. Deaths must be certified with causes listed. The subconscious assumption, born in the mentality of the Experiment, is that something has gone wrong. We will go to work on it. We will solve it.

The great therapeutic scheme that overarches the Experiment is one of manipulation and management. At many points it has unfortunate side effects, such as contributing to the population explosion, building up a genetic load in the population, reducing people to dehumanized mechanical entities, creating the spectre of unnecessary surgery, raising the moral ambivalence of life-prolonging or death-protracting treatments. Often manipulations yield dramatic and miraculous results. The auto accident victim whose body is pieced back together is such an example. The child with pulmonary pneumonia is pulled back from the brink. More often the case is not so dramatic. A disturbance, be it disease or accident, takes place. The body loses a little. The process runs its course. The trauma yields its full morbidity. We start now with what we have left and try to live again with diminished capacity, new limitations, but sustained hope and resolve.

Let me describe a scenario which will point up the unfortunate character of the Experiment. The senior physician leads his entourage of associates, residents, interns, and medical students down the hall of General Hospital. "We are going down the hall to see Mr. Smith," the chief says. "This is a classic case of Marfan's disease." "What about the old lady in this room?" a medical student asks as they pass a dimly lit room. "Oh, she's pretty well gone," says the chief resident. "Not much going on there."

In this not atypical situation are found all the ingredients of the Experiment. The modern teaching hospital is the "model" of the best place to be when you are sick. The scientific-technological orientation to disease is the operative interpretive model of what is going on for all except the patients, the night orderlies, and the family. But not the most revealing element in the scenario. Old Mrs. Jones is not interesting—she is dying. Mr. Smith down the hall holds out more teaching value, more exotic pathology, more scientific intrigue.

Mrs. Jones is coming to the great culmination of her life. She is about to discover what life is all about. In the glorious moments of the Tradition, family, friends, and neighbors would gather around her to experience vicariously this grand moment. Perhaps there would be words of counsel and wisdom—the dying person has many important things to say to us. In any case, it was considered the moment which gathered all preceding moments into a pattern of significance. Now with the tragic intellectual and attitudinal orientations of the Experiment, Mrs. Jones is a problem, an embarrasment, a symbol of medical and technical failure, an uninteresting, uninviting something to be avoided.

The Experiment is beginning to break down. It has lost its intellectual foundations as the earlier physicalistic reductionist

explanations of natural process are repudiated. The understandings of what causes and characterizes disease and health
are also opening up and becoming richer, more complex, more
mystery laden. A generation that has tried mechanistic and
manipulative therapeutics is driven to the realization that these
explanations are inadequate. Just as the spiritualistic healing of
the Tradition was doomed to collapse because of an inadequate view of creation and the body, so physicalistic
medicine faltered because of its reluctance to deal with the
dimension of the human spirit. We are therefore driven to
develop what might be called a Renovation of the Tradition. I
will turn to this new phase in the understanding of health and
disease after an illustration of the moral dilemma of the Experiment.

In 1925 William Faulkner introduced a figure and a theme
that was pivotal in his subsequent writing.[28] The sketch is called
"The Kingdom of God." Two bootleggers are trying to unload
some whiskey in a New Orleans alleyway. The dropoff is foiled
by the presence of a big, blubbering idiot brother of one of the
men. The retarded boy "with eyes blue as cornflowers" carries
a narcissus clutched tightly in one fist. While the mongol's
brother is trying to distract the policeman, the other bootleg-
ger violently slaps the helpless boy and breaks the stem of the
narcissus. The idiot howls a hoarse, inarticulate bellow which
draws a crowd along with the police. He continues to wail long
after his brother and the accomplice are arrested. Only when
the narcissus is mended with a stick an a bit of string is he stilled
and peace returns to his dramatic light-blue eyes.

The character is fully developed as Benjy six years later in
The Sound and the Fury. Faulkner gathers a rich literary tradition by painting the idiot with certain saintly and innocent
colors. The idiot is innocent in that he is not tainted with moral
wrong and is free from blame and built. The eye color, the
flower, and other symbols suggest innocence with a holy qual-

ity. The idiot is the special child of God. This outlook has always been a feature of the Tradition. The exceptional child has always provoked a particular awe and resultant devotion and staying power for the care he or she requires. In the primitive Gaelic tradition, for example, the Down's syndrome child is called the *duine le dia*, the person of God.

Faulkner entitled this sketch "The Kingdom of God." He likely had Mark 10:14–15 or Luke 18:17 in mind. The meaning of these passages is that only the "childlike" can enter the kingdom of God.[29] The wise, proud, and self-righteous have no spiritual inheritance. The simple, humble, poor, vulnerable and dependent are the special trust of God. They are the peculiar locus of his love and strength.

Now consider the profound effect on our moral consciousness when this myth is challenged by the new perception. The mood and ethos that we have labeled the Experiment have yielded the knowledge that the Down's syndrome child, the mongoloid, the holy idiot is simply the victim of a chromosomal anomaly, trisomy 21. This accounts for the multiple anomalies, including mental retardation, drawn eyes, and taut skin. Not only is the aberration known, but the knowledge and technology are now available to prevent the birth of the Down's syndrome child. Antenatal diagnosis of the fetus with amniocentesis can detect the presence of the extra chromosome, and selective abortion can see that the affected child is not born. New knowledge dispels former innocence and creates new ethical anguish. How are we to value the new life that is defected by mongoloid idiocy?

In 1959 the ancient aura of mystery surrounding mongolism was lifted when Jerome Lejeune and his associates in Paris discerned the chromosomal basis of this abnormality. It was this knowledge that made it possible in the early sixties to diagnose the fetus *in utero*. Like Oppenheimer and Einstein with the discoveries of nuclear secrets, Lejeune objected to this application of the knowledge as immoral and unethical. In an impassioned lecture to the American Society of Human Genetics he warned that joining the insights of prenatal diagnosis with selective abortion of abnormal fetuses would change the famous National Institutes of Health into a new "National Institutes of Death."

> I would come to very simple points now. When we discuss problems concerning adults and children, the National Institutes of Health is quite generally preferred. But when dealing with tiny fellows, expecially the not-yet-born, the National Institutes of Death finds some supporters. The reason for this divergence seems to lie in the question: Are they human or not? If already human, help and heal is the goal. If not yet human, discard and destroy is the solution. . . . My personal feeling is that we should elaborate our decison on scientific grounds . . . using all the scientific information we can gather.

> Let us take the example of trisomy 21, observed by amniocentesis. Looking at the chromosomes and detecting the extra 21 we say very safely, "The child who will develop here will be a trisomic 21." But this phrase does not convey all the information. We have also seen all the 46 other chromosomes and concluded that they were human, because if they had been mouse or monkey chromosomes, we would have noticed. Hence genetically speaking we have got two answers; first, here is a human being developing; second, he is affected by trisomy 21. All the discussion springs from the fact that some people note only the extra chromosome, and others look at the whole set.

> I have never believed myself the ensoulment theories (whether theological or materialistic) pretending that the developing thing in utero will become a man—some day, but is not yet human before a given step has been reached. Indeed this given step varies from specialist to specialist. But that is not the question. What seems obvious to me, from all we know about genetics, is simply this: if a fertilized egg is not by itself a full human being, it could never become a man, because something would have to be added to it; and we know that does not happen.[30]

This new knowledge also forces a change in our attitude. We cannot so readily see the child as a gift of God if we know the nature of the defect and have preventive capacity. Will we have the grace to care for the affected child that sustained parents in the past? Will we be able to surround the child with a symbolic aura that sees this being as special and precious? I recently discussed this issue with a family that had such a child. The father was a physician, and the entire family possessed a vibrant religious faith. Their outlook seemed to be typically human and fully natural. "We would not take anything for the experience, nor would we desire it again."

The capacity carried in the Experiment and the shift in attitude it precipitates drive us back to a theological understanding of the nature and meaning of the experience life brings. The ancient symbolic interpretation of the holy idiot was, in one sense, a rationalization of an enigmatic zone of experience over which we had no control. Like the bubonic plague before its complex etiology was known (*Pasturella pestis* bacillus, *Pulex irritans* fleas, rats, rancid water supplies, etc.), we could only chalk it up to the inscrutible will of God. Now that power to understand and control are delivered into our ken, we can no longer responsibly exercise this rationalization. In the midst of this new freedom, we can retain the Tradition's wisdom to gracefully accept what God gives. We will acknowledge that he has the power to transform darkness into light, tragedy into joy, weakness into power. We can still trust that he will also give us grace sufficient to every need and not test us beyond that which we are able to endure. But we will also sieze upon the capacities he has given us to more fully take advantage of the possiblities inherent in life. We will not crave illness because it is enobling, nor will we knowingly inflict suffering on others because it is good for the soul.

A rich Biblical theme comes into play at this point. Barnebas Ahern, the Roman Catholic scholar, has recently reviewed the biblical consideration of the Anawim, the humble and lowly,

God's special people.[31] The origin of the notion of the lowly as favored, which is the most vivid way that transcending value bears on the question of the exceptional and helpless, is found in the opening verses of Genesis, where God's spirit hovers over the void and darkness of the primeval waters. His Spirit brings Cosmos out of chaos, form from nothing (Genesis 1:2.) So with a collective people (Israel) and individuals (the weak, sick, and poor), he brings greatness out of nothing. Israel is born to an aged mother and father. Samuel is God's gift to a barren mother. In words that Mary, the mother of Jesus, will recall in The Magnificat, Anna exults:

> My heart hath rejoiced in the Lord; and my strength is exaulted in my God . . . because I rejoice in Thy salvation. . . . The Lord maketh poor and maketh rich; he humbleth and he exalteth. He raiseth up the needy from the dust, and lifteth up the poor from the dust, That he may sit with princes, and hold the throne of Glory (Samuel 2:1, 7).

Those who are contrite, broken, lowly, and bent down are the blessed of the Lord. They bear the spirit of *anawah*, poverty. God hears the affliction (*ani*) of his poeple (1 Samuel 1:11). The Anawim are those who inherit the Kingdom (Matthew 5:3–10). They stand with the Messiah at the threshold of the new age. Indeed, their broken existence welcomes the Kingdom. "The feeling of absolute dependence," writes Friedrich Schleiermacher, "is in and of itself God's co-presence in the self-consciousness."[32] The idiot Myshkin in Dostoevsky's great novel *The Idiot* is a gentle, innocent person who sees more clearly than the others, his penetrating perceptions undistorted by sham and pretense. Like Benjy, he becomes a moral compass, discerning truth in the midst of lies. In one great scene, the epileptic stands by a disgraced girl at whom the children are throwing stones and affirms her humanity, transforming hatred into care.

How can we synthesize the new empirical data with the deep truths of this artistic and biblical tradition? How can the Experiment and the Tradition be reconciled? Bishop John Morkovsky, the saintly scholar who shepherds the Houston-Galveston diocese, was recently asked to pray at the opening of the Jerry Lewis Telethon which raised money for research in muscular dystrophy. His prayer thanked God for the Anawim, the poor afflicted dear ones whom God places in the midst of our life to call us to faithfulness and humility. The prayer seemed to strike a sensitive judgment on these issues. We should not wish that God inflict some for our benefit. We who are healthy are thankful when we see the sick, the disabled, the poor. But we should not say, "there but for the grace of God go I." This would imply that God required the poor and afflicted to taunt the rich and those who do not need the physician. Should we not rather say that he can raise up power from nothing, strength from weakness, perfection from imperfection, incorruptible from corruptible?

While we live under the conditions of matter and time, our existence will be flawed. Devastating physical and mental anomalies will continue to afflict people through genetic and congenital as well as traumatic injury. We should work hard to prevent these injuries. We should strive to offset the deleterious effects of such injuries. We should create the conditions that will allow more children to be born healthy into a loving and supportive environment. But when the misfortune occurs, we should accept it as opportunity, as blessing, as the possibility to probe new dimensions of our being and unknown reaches of the mercy of God.

The mania for perfection and the impatience with pain and imperfection that characterize human life under the Experiment will make all the more necessary public policy protections of "abnormal" and weak lives.

At this point we can see the wisdom of the Judaic—and

subsequently Christian—notion of obligation to the weak, injured, and helpless. Those who codified the moral sense of Israel in the Levitical code had a vivid sense of the moral presence of Yaweh, who was no respecter of persons—who indeed was predisposed in mercy toward those who were "ana" (nothing). The theologians also looked at the natural human response, which seemed to be contempt and disregard for the afflicted. Out of this disparity the elaboration of divine law in cultic formulation was articulated. The compassion of God required that people bridle their natural disinclination to mercy and honor the being of their fellows—the neighbor, the stranger, the sick and helpless.

The best theology of health and disease will be a perspective where the genius of the Experiment is blended with the supernatural wisdom of the Tradition. This synthetic view I call the Renovation, and its development is discussed in the next chapter.

IV

The Renovation

———————◇———————

O, woman, you may keep the gold
The child we seek doesn't need our gold
On love alone he will build his kingdom
His pierced hand will hold no sceptre
His hallowed head will wear no crown
His might will not be built on your toil
Swifter than lightning he will soon walk among us
He will bring us new life
And receive our death.

—GIAN-CARLO MENOTTI, *Amahl and the Night Visitors*[1]

We live in the midst of a reformation, a revolution, a Renovation. All of these words suggest a recapitulation of something traditional, something basic. Psychologically speaking, we can see a certain affinity between the radical conservative and the radical liberal. In contrast to the bureaucrat, both radicals want change. The yearning to recover is much like the striving to discover. What is the Renovation I sense emerging in our understanding of health and disease?

Initially, it is characterized by a sense that the Experiment has, in part, proven detrimental. The Experiment's strengths have become its weaknesses. Its advances have created suffering; its successes have created new diseases. In many ways the Experiment has become counterproductive. It is part of a structural malaise. "Like time-consuming acceleration, stupefying education, self-destructive military defense, disorienting information or unsettling housing projects, pathological medicine is the result of industrial overproduction that paralyzes autonomous action."[2]

For example, our society, founded in the optimism of the European Enlightenment, while enjoying unprecedented and unparalleled biomedical progress, cannot be said to enjoy happiness, health, or well-being. The burden of morbidity is increasing. The obsession with health and sickness has intensified. The cost has burgeoned to the breaking point.

Yet at long last, we are beginning to sober up. We remember that health maintenance is a simple thing. It has to do with spiritual and social energies. Rather than medicalizing and consumerizing our existence further, we need to take initiatives for preventive medicine and self-care. We need to find ways to sustain health in one another through responsible use of the environment, mutual love, and fairness. We need to temper and contour strivings for physical perfection and immortality. We need to accept life and death as wise gifts from the hand of our Maker.

The Tradition was never a settled thing. There was always a straining forward, a desire to correct flaws. The great corrective influence was the response of people. There comes a time when we cannot accept conventional understandings. The Tradition was always being reformed. Likewise, the Experiment has been uneasy with itself. The factor of self-criticism has located flaws in the approach and hinted at ways to go beyond these weaknesses. A new sense of the meaning of health and disease is emerging. It would not be fair to call it a restoration; but we are witnessing a Renovation, in which certain features of the Tradition are being recovered. The Experiment is not being abandoned; we are merely building on the foundation it has fashioned while rejecting its unacceptable elements.

It is important to note that those possessed with sound

spiritual and moral values always affirm the enduring worth of the Tradition along with the positive possibility in the Experiment. Just as in the area of human justice the leaders who challenged the ecclesiastical and civil establishment were most often committed pastors and laymen, so in the realm of human health, physicians and pastors who fought against the ecclesiastical traditions which distorted the nature of mental illness did it in the name and power of religious faith. Gregory Zilborg states that the ideologies that oppressed the sick were not shattered by "apostates and freethinkers but by the pious and devout."[2] Jonathan Edwards, despite the erroneous caricatures to which he has been subjected, was a spirit deeply committed to the traditional sense of meaning and to the experimental emphasis of the new science. He died in Princeton after subjecting himself to the experimental smallpox innoculation. Cotton Mather, the first important figure in American medicine, pioneered smallpox vaccination, microbial theory, and preventive medicine—all in the spirit of religious faith— quite to the consternation of most physicians and the laity of eighteenth-century Boston. Benjamin Rush, who has been called the father of American psychiatry, was the kind of conserving, caring, and pioneering figure he was because he was a Quaker.

In seventeenth-century England, Thomas Browne attempted synthesis in his *Religio Medici*. Von Helmont's and other nineteenth-century German scientists sought deep affinities between medicine and philosophy. Today, leading humanists and medical scientists are committed to showing the essential compatability, indeed the mutual interdependence, of theological and ethical perceptions with emerging biomedical knowledge.[3]

All signs point to the fact that we are searching for a new synthesis of traditional and experimental insight. Let us look at the tentative directions beginning to appear in this renovated interpretation of the meaning of health and disease, wherein man is seen as measured being, disease is interpreted as plight and possibility, and health is perceived as wholeness.

MAN AS MEASURED BEING

Our fundamental understanding of human nature, our place in the world, and our transcendental character is being revised. Man is not microcosm or master. He is both. As René Dubos has reminded us, the notion of "reverence for nature [man as microcosm] is compatible with willingness to accept responsibility [man as master] for a creative stewardship of the earth"[4] (bracketed expressions mine). While previous eras and moods have seen people as fragments within or lords over nature, the emerging sense of the Renovation is that we are measured beings—husbandmen, stewards, creatures within the natural world who have unique responsibilities for the on-going building of the earth. We are creatures at once finite and infinite, bounded and unbounded.

The emergence of a new scientific outlook where deep mystery and complexity replace the simple physicalistic reductionism is the intellectual foundation for the revised sense of man as measure being. When Louis Pasteur located convincing evidence for the germ theory of the origin of infectious disease, he saw it not as an insight that reduced people even more to creatures whose lives could be explained in terms of physical forces and causation but rather the opening of new levels of infinity. On his election to the French Academy in 1822 he said:

> Positivism does not take into account the most important of positive notions, that of the infinite. . . . The human mind actuated by an invincible force, will never cease to ask itself what is beyond? I see everywhere the inevitable expression of the infinite in the world.[5]

Just as the concepts of indeterminacy and relativity have

released physics from the older mechanistic theories, so now developments in molecular biology have opened the dimensions of depth, mystery, even transcendence. Nobel laureate geneticist James Watson has shared in private conversation the image of the genetic code as a vast switchboard where certain processes are turned on and others remain turned off. It is as if an invisible hand moves along the switchboard and sets the basic processes of life in motion. Biologists Joshua Lederberg and Marshall Nirenberg have often invoked similar images. Unravelling the genetic code is gaining a glimpse of infinity.

In a provocative essay in *Nature,* biologist Gunther Stent argues that Salvador Dali was correct when he said in 1964, "The announcement of Watson and Crick about DNA . . . is for me the real proof of the existence of God." Stent proceeds to develop what he calls a "reminder of the transcendental basis of science," noting that discernment of the genetic code and developments in molecular biology give new credibility to Plato's monistic doctrine that "a single principle . . . not only regulates the course of the sun and the stars, but also prescribes to all creatures their proper behavior."[6] He goes on to say that Western intellectual thought remains muddled over the principal ethical derivative of this world view, the soul. The work of Thomas Szasz has raised the question of the nature, or even the existence, of mental illness. We are left with the possibility that "soul sickness" is only a species of material physical disorder. Stent suggests that perhaps only Eastern forms of thought, joined with scientific discoveries, can rescue us from the retreat of confidence that there is spirit in human nature, the natural world, and history.

Although Stent's point concerning the disregard for transcendence and soul in the modern mind may have force, it is uncertain whether philosophies of the East will have liberating influence. I believe that these dimensions will reappear in the bosom of Western thought. The Western tradition, which has so long had a materialistic, pragmatic concentration, will begin to affirm dimensions of depth and transcendence, if only for the reason that it is good science.

While in Eastern thought humanity is seen as integrated within the natural world and not radically distinct, the new sciences are driving us to a richer notion wherein human beings are unique, possessing infinite value while remaining part of the ecosphere. We are both angel and beast. We are the measure of things in our infinite qualities. Created in the image of God, we transcend space, time, and matter. But we are also measured beings. We are bounded by the limits of space and time.

Some authors have emphasized the unbounded character of humanity. Buckminster Fuller, in his ebullient optimism, has argued that we are bounded only by constrictions of intellect and imagination. We are capable of measures of creativity that we have not yet started to probe. We can utilize the resources of the earth frugally. We can contour the environment according to nature's own dynamic forms, thus enhancing our own life and beautifying the world.[7]

A renovated anthropology must affirm at once human grandeur and limitations. We can find fresh meaning in the words of Pico della Mirandola at the dawn of the Renaissance. The gods speak:

Neither a fixed abode nor a form that is thine alone nor any function peculiar to thyself have we given thee, Adam, to the end that according to thy longing and according to thy judgment thou mayest have and possess what abode, what form, and what functions thou thyself shalt desire. The nature of all other beings is limited and constrained within the bounds of laws prescribed by us. Thou constrained by no limits in accordance with thine own free will, in whose hand we have placed thee shalt ordain for thyself the limits of thy nature. . . . With freedom of choice and with honor, as though the maker and molder of thyself, thou mayest fashion thyself in whatever shape thou shalt prefer. Thou shalt have the power to degenerate into the lower forms of life, which are brutish. Thou shalt have the power, out of thy soul's judgment, to be reborn into the higher forms, which are divine.[8]

In the Renovation we see a convergence of the scientific notion that we are both grounded in and transcendent of nature and the Biblical sense of our responsible dominion. The overriding note that the Bible sounds is a strong affirmation of life. We are not to exult in weakness and suffering. Surely we are not to visit pain and destruction on ourselves and other creatures. We can desire pain, not in sado-masochism, but in the desire to overcome it in the affirmation of life. Kazoh Kitamori, in his great study *Theology of the Pain of God*, has shown that the strongest humanness and most authentic faithfulness develop when we meet pain head on and challenge it in the name of life. "We can conquer [pain] only when we seek it within ourselves and long for it. We can strengthen ourselves when we earnestly seek and desire pain to be a part of our nature."[9]

Whereas man as microcosm must concede to nature and man as master must override and consequently deny nature, man as measured being can accept suffering and transform it into an expression of strength and affirmation. Paul Tillich has reminded us that Christianity demands "that one accept suffering with courage as an element of finitude and affirm finitude in spite of the suffering that accompanies it."[10] We must be courageous today in our innovation, discovery, and creativity. We must be generous and compassionate in our ministrations to human need. The same courage should lead us to recognize, accept, and claim our limitations and death. "Not to accept an event which happens in the world is to wish that the world did not exist,"[11] writes Simone Weil. Not to accept what nature gives is fundamentally a denial of reality and a distrust of God. God is the "lover of life" (Wisdom of Solomon 11:26). The essence of his self-disclosure in the Old and New Testaments is that he loves; he affirms what we so easily reject. He affirms the worth of the poor, the weak, the sick. He affirms ourselves; he affirms reality. In this light, our facile rejections are denials of truth. "This wish is the state of sin. The person is curved in upon himself; pain has caused introversion. He has no future and can no longer love anything. He himself is everything; that is, he is dead."[12]

Our sense of measure allows us to accept the tension in our nature as healthy. We seek conquest and control. We acknowledge limitations which necessitate acceptance and acquiescence. Together these are reflections of our courageous glory.

In the renovated Tradition, though lord, we walk on the earth gently, with respect. There can no longer be the tinge of insecurity which sours our dominion into domination. We cherish life as it is given us. We guard it in ourselves and others. We honor the generations that have gone before us and take care for the generations that will come after. We come to accept thankfully the measure of life we have been given. We see it in the boundaries of appointed time and place. We accept the burden and opportunity of generativity and pass on life to a new generation. As Erik Erikson would contend, we give life to the future, both physically and spiritually.

Margery Shaw, an outstanding physician-geneticist in the Texas medical center, is now exploring the notion that the potential of life that resides in our gonads does not belong exclusively to us but to a future generation. As in the fiduciary relation, wherein parties hold property or wealth in trust, we are custodians for the life of a new generation. We are obliged for their sake to hold it in sacred trust. The specific implicatons of this view for genetic knowledge, conception control, antenatal diagnosis, child-bearing and rearing will demand thorough consideration. The general meaning of this orientation is that we are beings with possibilities and limitations. Our responsibility is intensified as knowledge grows. We are responsible for procreativity in demanding new ways. We are measured beings not so much in the sense of severe limitations that characterized former generations but in the sense of appropriateness and wisdom in our actions.

My great-great grandparents who came to Pennsylvania from Germany and Scotland were immigrants in a new land. Their life was limited by boundaries of knowledge, of food, of environment, of sickness and death. All of these limits, though still present, are diminished in their power over us. Limitations today are to some extent self-chosen. They come more from what in common sense we decide to be fitting and wholesome than from inevitability.

Perhaps the most challenging dimension of life where measured existence will be critical is our attitude toward death. Do we seek to defy not only natural but common-sense boundaries and seek to indefinitely prolong life? Do we deliberately seek to extend the life span? There is no doubt in my mind that gestures in pursuit of physical immortality and indefinite extension of the life span will become more credible as these become more theoretically feasible and technically possible. Will we continue to feel compelled to pursue the avenues of this quest by seeking to conquer cancer, developing the artificial heart, undertaking basic interventions at the genetic level, mechanizing and reduplicating life in a variety of ways with prosthetics? Or will we perhaps measure our life with more conscious determination and make the value-fraught decisions of who shall live and how we shall live?

Some of the ways that we will express our nature as measured beings will appear at the thresholds of birth and death. We will make determinations regarding the conception and birth of children with more knowledge and competence. We will more carefully exert quantity and quality controls over the children brought into the world. We are no longer passively subjected to the capricious forces of nature over which we have no control, nor will we feel so enraptured with our new-found knowledge and technique that we will attempt to "fabricate man." Rather, we will make meaningful choices and determinations within allotments and boundaries. Our decisions tempered by a renovated sense of appropriateness, we will make selective use of the new power. Potential technologies will range widely, offering many options for modifying the nature of our offspring and the experiences of conception and gestation. Recombinant DNA, changing certain genetic traits, may have the possibility of ameliorating gene-carried flaws and synthesizing new characteristics. If the tragedy of devastating illness like Tay-Sachs disease or other single-gene disorders can be alleviated, people will risk new techniques in order to maximize the chance of having healthy children. This will be particularly true for those who courageously wish to obviate the simple expedients of genetic screening, fetal diagnosis, and selective abortion. The same can be said for artificial donor insemination, prenatal diagnosis, in-vitro fertilization, extra-uterine gestation, and yet-to-come procedures. Where basic human yearnings—conceiving children, bearing healthy children, carrying children to term—are served, new powers will be utilized. When transhuman goals or interventions with offsetting side effects and prohibitive costs are proposed, people will decline in the name of qualitative life values. Medicare may give the party, but no one will come. People have already stopped lining up for heart transplants largely because of more realistic expectations. In the Renovation, we will exercise and modify our procreative powers, measuring our creativity with chosen limitations.

Likewise, at the end of life the Tradition and Experiment will begin to blend and provide us a sense of what is the best thing to do for the prolongation and preservation of life.

Should we introduce life supports—the respirator, intravenous feeding, blood transfusions, and so on—when there is no hope of recovery to meaningful existence? We will have the opportunity to make more conscious decisions regarding the time, setting, and manner that we die. Although death will always remain a mystery and terror and continue to come as a thief in the night, because of our technology we will have greater powers to bar the door, to delay its entrance.

Massachusetts General Hospital has recently established a permanent committee on optimum treatment of the hopelessly ill patient.[13] The mandate of the committee is to make discernments among patients regarding realistic hopes for recovery and then to correlate treatment intensity to the particular patient. Maximal therapeutic effort without reservation will be ordered in some cases, selective limitation of therapeutic measures in others. With some patients, the choice will be made to discontinue all therapy. This nuanced approach—as opposed to the blanket order for unconditional all-out treatment—is one example of our straining for a sense of what is appropriate in medical care. The program will be as vulnerable to abuses, mistakes, and the sheer weight of human ignorance as the present policy. But the personalized, particularized emphasis and the recognition that it is not always best *to* do all that we *can* do is a moral advance. This policy becomes a standardization of traditional clinical wisdom in the face of tendencies in the Experiment to be excessive, impersonal, and undiscriminating. It is Renovation.

In both birth and death we see the character of the Renovation unfolding. Primitive people knew that they should not do what they could not do. Experimental generations felt compelled to try everything they found the ability to do. The Renovation knows that there are some things we can do that we should not do. What is technologically feasible is not necessarily good. What is "technically sweet" need not be irresistable.

DISEASE AS PLIGHT AND POSSIBILITY

The intrusion of disease can no longer be seen simply as purposive in the sense that it conveys punishment or purification; nor is it accident, merely fortuitous and random. The Renovation sees plight and possibility in the experience of illness. This emerging way of looking at disease is, in some sense, a blend of Tradition and Experiment. We are responsible for our sickness and health in some ways. In others, we are not. In the Renovation sense of meaning, these questions are not especially helpful. We become sick. It is the common plight of the species. The important element is our response to the plight. How do we prevent disease, or experience it in the most meaningful way? How do we imbue it with possibility?

Our concepts of disease are now becoming more organismic and wholistic. The Experiment attempts to isolate specific natural causation. It seeks to localize in a part, an organ, a system, the disease entity. New knowledge is breaking down this model. Modern organismic, psychosomatic understanding of disease is antedated by the wholism of the biblical writers, again evidencing the fact that we are dealing with a recapitulation, not an invention.

The first transition step back from microorganic, fragmented medicine to wholistic medicine is one which sees the interrelation and interdependence of physical and mental function. The new science of biofeedback has shown the way in which all human systems interpenetrate. When we can monitor the activity of heart beat, galvanic skin response, stomach acid secretion, muscle tension, and so on, and change the physiological response by concentrated mind controls, we know that all systems—endocrine, central nervous, sympathetic, muscular—are intertwined in one wholistic sensation.

Much disease begins with a high specificity and localization and gradually takes on generalized systemic effect. The "black mole" melanoma is an extreme example of this. In other cases, a highly generalized disease expresses itself only later in localized symptoms. The gastric ulcer as sequel to organismic stress is an example of this situation. In both cases and both directions, disease and health are wholistic phenomena.

The mature Renovation sense of disease is that it is a systemic, ecological, natural-historical phenomenon. It is not so simple as to be something God has inflicted us with or even that he has sent us, although it is now more possible to give illness those interpretations than it was in the Experiment. We can no longer concentrate solely on the external vectors: the ontogenesis of disease, the germ etiology, the invasion of toxic and carcinogenic agents into the body, the diet and environmental stress to which we subject the body. There is truth in this perspective; indeed, it may be necessary causation, but it is not sufficient explanation for our illness. Nor is internal predisposition alone explanatory. Genetic predisposition is a strong factor. The immunological function of the body may be diminished or caught off-guard. The vulnerability of our organism may be increased by its being tired, stressed, or otherwise susceptible. Yet these predisposing factors alone will not suffice to explain the onset of illness.

It is very likely that a new sense of disease and health is emerging wherein the profound spiritual and moral dimensions, the environmental factors, the genetic predispositions, and the specific etiologic agents all seem to interplay, forming a wholistic context. Our nosology, or classification of diseases, must be comprehensive to be scientifically valid and therapeutically helpful.

Of the medical research in progress today, none seems to sketch the emerging sense of the nature of disease as well as Thomas Holmes' work on life events and the onset of illness. The phenomenon that Holmes seeks to describe, the hunch he proposes to explore with empirical investigation, has always been known by literature as well as by the perceptive physician. "It is changes that are chiefly responsible for diseases," writes Hippocrates, "especially the great changes, the violent alterations both in the seasons and in other things."[14]

Thomas Mann writes:

> His father and mother he had barely known: they had both dropped away in the brief period between his fifth and seventh birthdays; first the mother. . . . The father, Herman Castorp, could not grasp his loss. He had been deeply attached to his wife, and not being the strongest himself, never quite recovered from her death. His spirit was troubled; he shrank within himself; his benumbed brain made him blunder in his business, so that the firm of Castorp and Son suffered sensible financial losses; and the next Spring, while inspecting warehouses on the windy landing-stage, he got inflammation of the lungs. The fever was too much for his shaken heart and in five days, notwithstanding all Dr. Heidekind's care, he died.[15]

Somerset Maugham relates the same truth in *The Summing Up*:

> My father . . . went to Paris and became solicitor to the British Embassy. . . . After my mother's death, her maid became my nurse. . . . I think my father had a romantic mind. He took it into his head to build a house to live in during the summer. He bought a piece of land on top of a hill at Suresnes. . . . It was to be like a villa on the Bosphorus and on the top floor it was surrounded by loggias. . . . It was a white house and the shutters were painted red. The garden was laid out. The rooms were furnished, and then my father died.[16]

The question of what accounts for illness—why me?—is a perennial human query and quandary. Our interpretations have moved through the primitive, classical, and experimental stages. We have seen illness due to displeasure of the gods, imbalance of "humours," germ theory, and now an amplified physicalistic etiology where, in addition to infectious agents, flawed genes, trauma, tumors, poisons, and imbalances in the blood constituents are instrumental.

We now know that vulnerability and resistance to disease are extremely important variables. When Hong Kong flu appears, some succumb, others do not. Some are hospitalized. A few even die. Others experience nothing more than stomach cramps or diarrhea. What is resistance? People in excellent physical condition have coronaries and die. Many frail and sedentary folk become octogenarians. Mental attitude plays a part, but people in superb mental health often experience excessive disease. The hypochondriacal complainer often outlives his children.

Some authors have suggested life-style and life events as key factors. This line of evidence has shaped a new sense, which may be called an ecological interpretation of disease. Life is becoming a frantic race for many contemporary people. Society moves from one crisis to the next with the underlying malaise of insecurity, nuclear threat, unemployment, energy, and economic uncertainty becoming chronic. We are always moving and relocating. We are bombarded with experiential overload that threatens to break us.

Early in this century, Adolf Meyer, professor of psychiatry at Johns Hopkins, saw this new life-style emerging and began to keep "life charts" on his patients. These brief biographies vividly depicted the fact that people tended to get sick around the times when clusters of major events occurred in their lives. The horse and buggy days were disappearing and the ancient advice of Lao Tse—"Never go far from your home or get in anything with wheels"—went unheeded.

The idea that there are contextual and life-style factors involved in the onset of illness is, of course, not new. The ancients were very aware of this dimension. Hippocrates, for example, knew the triadic context of disease shaped by environment, disposition or temperment, and humoural imbalance. Although the Experiment in some ways undervalued it, the concept has regained currency in recent years. Harold G. Wolff, professor of neurology and psychiatry at Cornell University Medical College, studied intensively the life settings and emotional states surrounding many illnesses.[17] Thomas Holmes, a colleague of Wolff at Cornell, and his collaborators looked at people who have become sick and asked what significant life changes occurred in the preceding two years. The diseases Holmes followed included infectious and parasitic, psychosomatic, neoplastic, allergic, psychiatric, cardiovascular, neuroendocrinological, musculoskeletal, and other traumatic disorders. Patients around the world who experienced these problems examined their preceding months' experience and quantified what Holmes calls "life-change units." The inference, indeed, the clear implication, of the study is that a human being becomes ill when a burden of life-changing events accumulates that overwhelms the person's ability to cope with change. The experiences, listed below, are both tragic and unpleasant, happy and pleasant. They all entail a disruption of normal life-course rhythm, a break in accustomed equilibrium. They are disturbances in the customary patterns and routines that our lives regularly follow.

LIFE EVENTS SCALED IN DESCENDING ORDER OF SIGNIFICANCE

Death of spouse
Detention in jail
Divorce
Death of close family member
Major personal injury or illness
Marriage
Marital separation
Being fired from work
Major change in health of family member

Sex difficulties
Retirement from work
Major business readjustment
Pregnancy
Change to different line of work
Marital reconciliation
Death of close friend
Mortgage loan foreclosure
Son or daughter leaving home
Mortgage loan of $10,000 or more
In-law troubles
Major change in financial state
Major change in responsibility at work
New member to family
Outstanding personal achievement
Wife starting or ceasing work
Major change in living conditions
Troubles with boss
Minor violations of law
Revision of personal habits
Mortgage loan of less than $10,000
Major change in work hours or conditions
Beginning or end of formal schooling
Major change in arguments with spouse
Change to new school
Major change in sleeping habits
Major change in eating habits
Change in residence
Major change in recreation
Major change in social activities
Major change in family get-togethers
Vacation
Major change in church activities
Christmas

These life events are weighted in terms of how dramatically they throw off the normal life pattern. The death of a spouse may provide such profound disruption that it receives forty-three points. The Christmas season, though perhaps a happy time, provides sufficient distortion to normal schedule and mood that it rates one point. If in a two-year period a person accumulates 400 points—by experiencing major illness, being divorced, losing a job, having a mortgage foreclosed, and so forth—there is a high likelihood that he or she will become sick. There may be exceptions to the pattern. Some, like Job, can bear great tragic burdens to prove their faithfulness. Others may have extraordinary coping ability which allows them to accumulate great numbers of points without breaking down and becoming ill. However, the hypothesis that life events cluster significantly in the two-year period preceding the onset of disease is borne out by research.

> The findings from this study suggest the possibility that the greater the magnitude of the life crisis, the greater the probability the involved subjects' psychophysiologic activation will result in tissue, organ, and body system dysfunction. When so affected, a person may become vulnerable to available pathogens that under conditions of less life change could not overcome body resistance.[18]

The importance of Holmes' work is to restore a sense of pattern to the meaning we bring to disease. Illness is part of a broad fabric of experience which contains predictable and unpredictable threads. We are able to contribute positively to the maintenance of health. Yet a vast area remains outside our control.

We can work for an environment and life-style that are conducive to health and in many ways guard our health. Yet disease will intrude into human life and death will take its toll. We may wish to eat, drink, and be merry for tomorrow we die; or we may wish to refrain and lead a cautious and sensible life and die the day after tomorrow.

We see now that we are coming to accept a restored interpretation of the meaning of disease. Elements of the Tradition are being recovered. The ecological setting of illness and health is reaffirmed. Certain dimensions of human responsibility in the onset and course of sickness are reemphasized. The spiritual and moral character of illness, not in the sense of causation and blame, but in terms of plight and possibility, is again highlighted. We can even recover the wisdom of the demonic or diabolic theory of disease causation. Rollo May writes:

> The daimonic is any natural function which has the power to take over the whole person. Sex and eros, anger and rage, and the craving for power are examples. The daimonic can be either creative or destructive and is normally both. When this power goes awry and one element usurps control over the total personality, we have "daimon possession," the traditional name through history for psychosis.[19]

The devil in Christian thought is seen to be the intermediate power, greater than the human, less than God. Since nature is spiritual and not just flat, there are transcending powers which, despite our lack of control, remain under God's control. This realm of spirit has been called the demonic, or the devil. Satan, or the realm of the demonic in Biblical understanding, is the total realm of experience that subjects us to death. The New Testament speaks of "principalities and powers" (Romans 8:38; Ephesians 3:10). Frequently, the richness of our symbolic life has led us to personify this spiritual power. In the New Testament and subsequent history, demon possession, or demonmania, is frequently seen as the explanatory factor in disease. The genius of the insight is the fact that those forces that enslave or consume are indeed diabolic; they split and tear apart rather than integrate (make symbolic) our existence.

The literal vision of the concrete representation of evil came to an absurd conclusion in the identification and burning of witches. This mood in Medieval and Puritan Christianity is an aberration, a constriction in our sense of the demonic. The lasting meaning of the demonic is in its reference to that gap between the human will and God's control. There are evils and afflictions which we cannot control. They cannot be attributed to the divine, as he has revealed his character: loving and benevolent. Therefore we label them demonic. The powers may be seen as God's allowance. The devil is not the direct expression of God's will. It is spiritual power, born in rebellion, intensified by human sin, shaped in the dimension of freedom that God allows. These powers are being stripped of their energy in God's redemptive purchase of nature and history. All enemies shall be put under his feet; even death loses its sting (1 Corinthians 15). Ultimately death is subject to him.

HEALING AS WHOLENESS

Some features of the traditional understanding of healing are also proving to have enduring value. In the ancient cultures of Egypt and Asia as well as those of Greece and Rome, physicians practiced spiritual healing as an essential dimension of bodily healing. The Asclepian cult of medicine, for example, was a priesthood which practiced faith healing based on dreams. The central therapeutic impulse of the cult was the healing power of the god.

The Asclepian temples were sanctuaries where wholistic diets, purifying waters and baths, anointments, counseling, and meditation were all seen as elements of healing. In the medical ministrations in the sanctuary, the environment was crucial. The religious aura evoked the body's own therapeutic action as well as the healing visitation of the gods.

A parallel tradition which emphasized medical interventions was also followed by the Asclepiads. The wandering, sandal-clad doctors treated patients with the prevailing physiological knowledge and therapeutics, using drugs, surgery, and other regimens. This tradition, which is the root of Hippocratic medicine, also grew to flower into the Experiment.

Now we can begin to see the joining of the two streams of Asclepian wisdom: the blending of Tradition and Experiment. We can see the necessity of holding *Hygeia* and *Panacea* together. Preventive and interventive medicine combine to fashion the new sense of therapeutics. The enriched understanding of therapeutics is evoked by an emerging sense of the wholistic nature of healing.

A gracious and magnificent marble head of Christ adapted from a bust of Asclepius symbolized the way that Greek naturalism and Christian theism synthesized into a new wholistic view of health. In the renovated sense of the meaning of health and disease, this wholistic interpretation prevails.

The first significant figure in American medicine is generally considered to be the Reverend Dr. Cotton Mather.[20] A clerical physician, he practiced medicine as a part of his pastoral work. He apprenticed his daughter Katy, the first American woman to seriously study medicine. Wholism was the essence of his theological medicine. He saw the brilliance of the human organism in disease and healing to be its natural responsiveness under supernatural impulses. Mather's thought on the meaning of sickness and healing was built on the foundation of a providential theology. Nothing in nature transpires outside of the divine will. God commits his governance of the natural world to secondary causes, which people are invited to study, understand, and interpose in the service of life. Yet human intervention should be cautious, focused on the demonic misappropriations of nature's laws, affirming divine patterns. This struggle is vividly described as Mather grapples with his own son's demand to be inoculated against smallpox. The following passage from Mather's diary relates his anguish whether to acquiesce or intervene in the face of providence as he searches for an ethical response.

[May] 26 [1721]. The grievous Calamity of the Smallpox has now entered the Town. The Practice of conveying and suffering the Smallpox by Inoculation, has never been used in America, nor indeed in our Nation, But how many Lives might be saved by it, if it were practised?

[June] 13. What shall I do? what shall I do, with regard unto Sammy? He comes home, when the Smallpox begins to spread in the Neighbourhood; and he is lothe to return unto Cambridge. I must earnestly look up to Heaven for Direction.

[July] 16. At this Time, I enjoy an unspeakable Consolation. I have instructed our Physicians in the new Method used by the Africans and Asisticks, to prevent and abate the Dangers of the Smallpox, and infallibly to save the Lives of those that have it wisely managed upon them. The Destroyer, being enraged at the Proposal of any Thing, that may rescue the Lives of our poor People from him, has taken a strange possession of the People on this Occasion. They rave, they rail, they blaspheme; they talk not only like Ideots but also like Franticks, And not only the Physician who began the Experiment, but I also am an Object of their Fury.

[August] 1. Full of Distress about Sammy; He begs to have his Life saved, by receiving the Smallpox, in the way of Inoculation, whereof our Neighbourhood has had no less than ten remarkable Experiments; and if he should after all dy by receiving it in the common Way, how can I answer it? On the other Side, our People, who have Satan remarkably filling their Hearts and their Tongues, will go on with infinite Prejudices against me and my Ministry, if I suffer this operation upon the Child.

15. My dear Sammy, is now under the Operation of receiving the Smallpox in the way of Transplantation. The Success of the Exper-

iment among my Neighbours, as well as abroad in the World . . . [has] made me think, that I could not answer it unto God, if I neglected it.

25 d. VI m. Friday. It is a very critical Time with me, a Time of unspeakable Trouble and Anguish. My dear Sammy, has this Week had a dangerous and threatening Fever come upon him, which is beyond what the Inoculation for the Smallpox has hitherto brought upon my Subjects of it. In this Distress, I have cried unto the Lord; and He has answered with a Measure of Restraint upon the Fever. The Eruption proceeds, and he proves pretty full, and has not the best sort, and some Degree of his Fever holds him. His condition is very hazardous.

[September] 5. Sammy recovering Strength, I must not earnestly putt him on considering, what he shall render to the Lord! Use exquisite Methods that he may come Gold out of the Fire.

[November] 19. Certainly it becomes me and concerns me, to do something very considerable, in a way of Gratitude unto GOD MY SAVIOR, for the antonishing Deliverance, which He did the last Week bestow upon me, and upon what belong'd unto me.[21]

Note how reliance on God and human creativity are interrelated both in the decision to treat and in the response to recovery. The perspectives of the Tradition and the Experiment intertwine into a wholistic sense of meaning. Today these classic meanings of health and healing are regaining currency. *Salvus*, salve, salvation; *Heil*, *Heiligkeit*, hale, whole, holy—the words all connote completeness, integrity. Health is not only being in equilibrium, it is being at peace. We can be caught up in suffering and death and at the same time in the profoundest transformation of healing. "I think science more and more is going to be giving its attention to finding ways whereby humanity can live at peace with itself and nature," Loren Eisely reflected on the renewed sensibility of the Renovation.[22] Our passions for control and conquest are being contoured into meaningful goals which are in the service of humanity and human values. Jürgen Moltmann expresses the same view: "Just because biomedical progress elicits hopes and yet does not contain a guarantee of happiness, it must be guided by a humane ethic which ought to lead from the struggle for existence to peace in existence."[23]

Indeed, the struggle for existence may be a part of peace in existence. Healing means restoration to wholeness. When we are sick, we are subjected for awhile to the threats of pain, abandonment, and extinction. Great cleavages open in the body and spirit, and the abyss appears. We are restored as the agency inflicting disease is removed, as body and soul have a chance to mend, as we are reincorporated into the community. We do not recover some former perfect state of well-being but rather learn to live in spite of increasing maladies and increased frailty.

Healing can be viewed somewhat in the spirit of Erik Erikson. We grow into adulthood, old age, and death. There are attendant difficulties, joys, and opportunities at each stage of life. Fulfillment for the young is to grow and change and discover the new. Fulfillment in old age is found in imparting wisdom, relaxing while watching from a distance the blessings of our generativity—the children and grandchildren—and anticipating life's culmination in peace. Healing is thus a process of becoming our possibility, our destiny.

The movement toward wholism opens again the possibility, indeed the necessity, of seeing disease and health in a theological frame. A new sense of the meaning of illness and well-being as well as refreshed commitments to care for each other in life and death are possible as we recover the themes of creation and redemption.

Theology today is calling into question the view of God as creator and sustainer that we have inherited in Western Culture. The static-being notion that prevails in Greco-Roman religion is challenged in the light of the Lord of nature and history and the Yearning Savior of humanity that we meet in the faith of Old and New Testament communities. The sense we give to human beings and their experience is derivative of our image of and relationship to God. The reality of God is indeed the context wherein we shape our sense of being and destiny. The meaning of disease, health, and death are developed within this reality.

Western theology was shaped in the crucible of Greek thought, wherein God is seen as apathetic being. God is removed from the constraints of time and space. He is incapable of suffering. The strength of this metaphysical and ethical view enabled it to endure in Christian theology without the censure of heresy. It remains a strain in Plato and Aristotle and the derivative work of Augustine and Aquinas, despite their loyalty to the agapic and pathetic God of Scripture, which is dominant. *Apatheia* is a force within Protestant and Catholic orthodoxy and the modern scholastic faith that has sought to systematize the dynamic insights of biblical faith. God as *actus purus* is perfect being. He needs nothing. He cannot suffer. Anger, passion, and envy are stripped away as divine attributes—a refinement, perhaps, over primitive faiths. But qualities of love, compassion, and mercy are also lost. In this spirit human beings can only be imperturbable, passive, and stoic in the experience of health and disease.

Abraham Heschel, in controversy with Hellenic Judaism and the derivative thought of Maimonides and Spinoza, reclaimed for us the prophetic proclamation of God as pathetic being. The prophets did not have a picture or idea of God. God gathers his people into his being, his situation. God is affective and affected. He is affected by events, by what happens to his people, by pain and suffering. He is interested and involved in what happens with his loved ones. The *Anawim,* the dear ones who innocently suffer, are particularly precious to Him (Amos 2:6–7; Zephaniah 3:12, Isaiah 55:1, 2). His Servant suffers with us and for us.

God's sympathy with us is the impulse for our sympathy. He identifies with us in life and death. He draws us into the rich dimensions of his life in the plight and possibility of our disease. Our frailty, sickness, and death are caught up through his redeeming weakness and transformed into wisdom and power.

In a telling critique of the sado-masochistic strain in Western theology, Dorothee Sölle argues that the biblical tradition is distorted when we fashion God into a being who inflicts pain in order to test, try, or punish us. The God and Father of Jesus Christ does not crucify his Son. He gave his Son, delivered him up unto death, so that through belief we should be healed. God does not need to render us sick and abject that he might rule; his power is not posited on our impotence. His might is not built upon our toil. He gives us life with newness and freshness. He receives our death and we die into life.

The pathetic way of life prompted by our identification with the Living God is one that conflicts with the prevailing apathy. Sölle describes it:

> One wonders what will become of a society in which certain forms of suffering are avoided gratuitously, in keeping with middle-class ideals. I have in mind a society in which: a marriage that is perceived as unbearable quickly and smoothly ends in divorce: after divorce no scars remain; relationships between generations are dissolved as quickly as possible, without a struggle, without a trace; periods of mourning are "sensibly" short; with haste the handicapped and sick are removed from the house and the dead from the mind. If changing marriage partners happens as readily as trading in an old car on a new one, then the experiences that one had in the unsuccessful relationship remain unproductive. From suffering nothing is learned and nothing is to be learned.[24]

This life-style is not only superficial and sick, it removes us from the deeper reaches of the human experience. God is at work in the world, suggested Bonhoeffer, where human sufferings signal the presence of Christ. "God becomes immanent," says Kitamori, "in these realities of pain."[25]

The experience of childbirth provides one illustration among many of human sensibility moving full circle from Tradition to Experiment to Renovation. Until the end of the nineteenth century, midwives assisted mothers in natural childbirth at home. Then in Germany and France, the specialty of obstetrics developed, and childbirth became a clinical process. Under this influence, the American specialty of OB–Gyn developed, and childbirth was transferred to hospitals. As doctors became enamored with powers of technical management of this great human experience, cesarean section became a fashionable mode of childbirth. In the early 1930s, nearly one fourth of deliveries studied in New York City and Philadelphia involved operative procedures.[26] Some preferred to speak of pregnancy as a disease and delivery as a medical problem. The German tradition of limited analgesia gave way to deep anesthesia, which served not only to alleviate pain but also to obliterate consciousness and participation as well. Gradually, partial blocks enabled mothers to participate more in the grand experience. Today thousands of couples choose the method of Lamaze natural childbirth in order to fully participate in the painful joy of the moment of birth. The benefit of the hospital is recognized. The antiseptic environment and the armamentarium of skills for crises that might develop are welcomed, but the humanness of the event is retained as father and mother together greet life's miracle. One day childbirth may be moved back into the home. If so, it will find some way to take the blessed technical abilities of modern medicine (Experiment) together with the rich natural meanings (Tradition) and fashion a new sensible synthesis (Renovation).

The transition I have described from Tradition to Experiment to Renovation has been an especially difficult transaction for people working in the healing professions. The ministries of medicine, nursing, and pastoral care, along with the variety of vitally essential helping ministries, have had their knowledge base so enriched that no one can feel competent except in a very specific area. The derivative therapeutic arts have also been opened as diversity, not uniformity, of treatment has become the rule. Now, as if the loss of intellectual and practical underpinnings of the professions were not enough, there has ensued a loss of vocational sense and an identity crisis in all the major healing professions. One author has sensitively referred to the condition as that of the "wounded healer."[27] I would refer this operational and intellectual crisis back to the collapse of a theological framework within which disease and health can be understood.

Robert Jay Lifton, the psycho-historian, has noted that everyone today experiences historical dislocation, fragmented ideology, and search for immortality.[28] This generalized disorientation is acute in the health professional. Henri Nouwen is in agreement with Lifton's argument that the collapse of the sense of immortality and the derivative quest for enduring value are at the heart of the modern malaise. The sense of immortality "represents a compelling, universal urge to maintain an inner sense of continuity over time and space, with the various elements of life. It is man's way of experiencing his connection with all human history."[29]

In these words, Lifton speaks in a renovating spirit. When immortality is seen in terms of linking the pieces—past, present, and future—together in a meaningful pattern, it is wholesome. Very frequently, however, the quest for immortality is seen as a yearning for discontinuity, for a radical break from the past and present. In our discussion of the Nordic "master" mentality, we hinted at the distorted grasping towards immortality that is basic to the dominating mythology.

More meaningful today in the light of our situation, our theology, and human need all around us, would be a theology of identification and humility. A true sense of transcending spiritual value will lead us to deeply participate in the anguish of our world and the presence everywhere of the suffering.

Nouwen uses the image of a wounded healer. Perhaps the greatest opportunity present in the new crisis is that, stripped of our pretense and authority, we can now minister to one another in the only way that has ever really counted, as servants. The physician has the opportunity to attend patients through illness, to watch with them and lend assistance as the body and mind heal themselves. The physician has, with the pastor, the privilege of accompanying people into the great crises of birth, suffering, healing, and death. Nouwen characterizes the broken and wounded healer as the hospitable companion.

> Hospitality . . . gives us insight into the nature of response to the human condition of loneliness. Hospitality is the virtue which allows us to break through the narrowness of our own fears and to open our houses to the stranger, with the intuition that salvation comes to us in the form of a tired traveler. Hospitality makes anxious disciples into powerful witnesses, makes suspicious owners into generous givers. . . . Like the Semitic nomads, we live in a desert with many lonely travelers who are looking for a moment of peace, for a fresh drink and for a sign of encouragement so that they can continue their mysterious search for freedom.[30]

We learned of the blessedness of hospitality in Bubba's final hours. "That damn towel! That damn basin!" he cried in the midst of excruciating pain near his death. "That's what it's all about!" "Come ye blessed of my father, inherit the kingdom prepared for you from the foundation of the world: for I was . . . sick and ye came unto me . . ." (Matthew 25:34–40, KJV).

V

Conclusion

———————◇———————

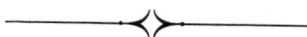

I have attempted to recount the history, to paint the moods of our human attempt to make sense out of disease and health. My thesis, simply stated, is that a perennial stream of wisdom flows from the beginnings of humanity even into our post-modern age. A strong undercurrent of resistance to some aspects of the wisdom tradition has always been present. It creeps to the surface in the era of the Experiment and mixes in an indissoluble way with the Tradition stream, releasing a new upsurge with a new character. This synthesis I have called the Renovation.

Lest I leave the impression that we are powerless victims of an inevitable process that is working itself out, let my conviction be clear that we can direct the course of our conceptualization and concrete actions in the realm of health and disease. I feel that it is now demanded of us that we formulate a philosophy of medicine, a theology of health and disease—what Jonas Salk calls a "metabiology." We must decide the values we will pursue in the realm of biomedical research and health care and set out resolutely to realize those values.

Individual growth and development is microcosmic of the common experience of humankind. There are continuities in life with perennial impulses to innovation. Our genius, indeed, is the ability we possess to imagine the novel and test it, discard the aberrations, and draw the positive elements inward to enrich the central core of our essence and growth.

We are now, as always, in this upbuilding process. It is dramatic and rapid in our time. Because of our growing knowledge and technology, we experience the novel possibility with such intensity that we are not sure what constitutes that enduring center. The experimental mood entails a suspension of what was once held to be normative. This is true not only in science but in moral values and religion. Yet after the initial suspension of the norm to test the novel, the traditional reasserts itself because the new situation demands it for its own completeness.

Our culture stands at the threshold of great innovations in the area of health and disease. We shall rapidly develop the power to make profound modifications over what once were seen to be the natural, inevitable, and sacrosanct thresholds of birth and death. Our skills will make possible profound alterations during life's course, powers that entail nothing less than the ability to change human nature. We will be enticed by the new possibility and repelled by its challenge; but finally we will edge forward, straining to retain the inherited sense of what is good together with the modifications of that wisdom carried in the new opportunity. To sustain a creative tension between the enduring and the *ex*otic remains the ethical mandate.

> As Jesus went along, he saw a man who had been blind from birth. His disciples asked him, "Rabbi, who sinned, this man or his parents, for him to have been born blind?" "Neither he nor his parents sinned," Jesus answered; "he was born blind so that the works of God might be displayed in Him" (John 9:1–3).

Notes

I. INTRODUCTION

1. For recent expositions of the theodicy question, see John Hick, *Evil and the God of Love* (London: Macmillan, 1966); and Albert Outler, *Who Trusts in God; Musings on the Meaning of Providence* (Oxford: Oxford University Press, 1968).
2. Charles Raven, *Science, Medicine and Morals: A Survey and a Suggestion* (London: Hodder and Stoughton, 1959), p. 11.
3. Kenneth Vaux, *Biomedical Ethics* (New York: Harper & Row, 1974).
4. Walther Riese, *The Conception of Disease* (New York: Philosophical Library, 1953), p. 1.
5. Ernest Becker, *The Denial of Death* (Glencoe, Ill.: Free Press, 1965), p. 2.
6. Numerous studies point up the surprising pervasiveness of spiritual and moral ideation as patients experience disease and healing. See, for example Seward Hiltner, *A Preface to Pastoral Theology* (Nashville: Abingdon Press, 1958); and Renée Fox, *Experiment Perilous: Physicians and Patients Facing the Unknown* (Glencoe, Ill.: Free Press, 1959).
7. Galen, "The Use of Limbs," Section 3, *On the Natural Faculties* (Cambridge, Mass.: Harvard University Press, Loeb Classical Library, 1948).

II. THE TRADITION

1. Eliot Wiginton, ed., *The Foxfire Book I* (Garden City, N.Y.: Doubleday, 1972), p. 29.
2. René Dubos, *Man Adapting* (New Haven, Conn.: Yale University Press, 1965), p. 35.
3. Morris Leikind, "Colonial Epidemic Diseases," *Southern Medicine*, December 1975, pp. 32, 33.
4. Bert Kaplan and Dale Johnson, "The Social Meaning of Navajo Psychopathology and Psychotherapy" in *Magic, Faith and Healing*, ed. Ari Kiev (New York: Free Press, 1964), p. 206.
5. Michael Banton, ed., *Anthropological Approaches to the Study of Religion*

(London: Avistock Publications, 1966), pp. 19ff. See also Kiev, *Magic, Faith and Healing*.

6. Phillis Garlick, *Man's Search for Health* (London: The Highway Press, 1952), p. 99.

7. Garlick, p. 92.

8. Garlick, p. 96.

9. Garlick, p. 104.

10. Much research needs to be done on the health-nurturing aspects of religious faith and life style. See, for example, Kenneth Vaux, "Religious Beliefs and Health Behavior," *Preventive Medicine*, 5, no. 4 (December 1976), pp. 331–347.

11. S. J. McMillen, *None of These Diseases* (Old Tappan, N.J.: Fleming H. Revell Co., 1968).

12. Max Weber, *Ancient Judaism* (New York: Free Press, 1952).

13. Price Cobbs and William H. Grier, *Black Rage* (New York: Bantam, 1969), p. 24.

14. Jürgen Moltmann, *The Crucified God* (New York: Harper & Row, 1974), p. 4.

15. Emil Fackenheim, *God's Presence in History* (New York: New York University Press, 1970), p. 5.

16. Kaspar Naegele, *Health and Healing* (San Francisco: Jossey-Bass, 1970), p. 28.

17. Riese, p. 93.

18. Garlick, p. 154.

19. Karl Barth, *Church Dogmatics IV–II* (Edinburgh: T & T Clark, 1958), pp. 485–486.

20. C. S. Lewis, *The Problem of Pain* (London: Centenary, 1940), p. 81.

21. J. Eric Thompson, "Sixteenth and Seventeenth Century Reports on the Chol Mayas," *American Anthropologist* 40 (1938), p. 602.

22. John Wesley, *Primitive Remedies* (Santa Barbara, Calif.: Woodbridge Press), pp. 9–14© 1973 by Howard B. Weeks. Originally published as *The Primitive Physick* in 1751.

23. Wesley, p. 62.

24. G. Dock, "The Primitive Physic of Rev. John Wesley: A Picture of Eighteenth Century Medicine," *JAMA* 64: 629–638, 1915.

25. Oliver W. Holmes, cited in T. R. Harrison, *Principles of Internal Medicine* (New York: McGraw-Hill, 1958), p. 632.

26. Wesley, p. 5.

27. Wesley, p. 13.

28. Wesley, p. 14.

29. Wesley, pp. 9–11.

30. Wesley, p. 22.

31. Ivan Illich, *Medical Nemesis* (New York: Pantheon, 1976), pp. 130, 131.

III. THE EXPERIMENT

1. From *Man of La Mancha* by Dale Wasserman and Joe Darion (New York: Random House, 1966). Reprinted by permission of the publisher.
2. Robert Morse, quoted in the *New York Times*, October 21, 1975.
3. Joseph Quinlan, quoted in the *New York Times*, October 21, 1975.
4. Pierre Teilhard de Chardin, *Letters to Two Friends* (New York: New American Library, 1968), pp. 78, 79.
5. Osborne Segerberg, *The Immortality Factor* (New York: Dutton, 1974), pp. 9, 10.
6. Quoted in Segerberg, p. 10.
7. Riese, p. 5.
8. C. G. Jung, *The Psychogenesis of Mental Disease* (New York: Pantheon, 1960), p. 211.
9. Garlick, p. 211.
10. Riese, p. 83.
11. William Osler, *The Old Humanities and the New Science* (New York: Houghton Mifflin, 1920), pp. 2ff.
12. David Mechanic, "Health and Illness in Technological Societies," *Hastings Center Studies*, vol. 1, no. 3, 1973, p. 9.
13. Eric Kahler, in *The Germans*, ed. Robert Kimber and Rita Kimber (Princeton, N.J.: Princeton University Press, 1974), p. 28.
14. Representative literature includes Hans Reichenback, *The Rise of Scientific Philosophy* (Berkeley, Calif.: University of California Press, 1951), E. A. Burtt, *The Metaphysical Foundations of Modern Science* (Garden City, N.Y.: Doubleday, 1955); Floyd W. Matson, *The Broken Image: Man, Science and Society* (Garden City, N.Y.: Doubleday, 1964).
15. Gotthard Booth, "Health From the Standpoint of the Physician," in *The Church and Mental Health*, ed. Paul Maves (New York: Scribner's, 1953), pp. 3ff.
16. Illich, p. 195.
17. Niels Bohr, *Atomic Physics and Human Knowledge* (New York: Wiley, 1958), p. 95.
18. John Hermann Randall, *The Making of the Modern Mind*, rev. ed. (New York: Houghton Mifflin, 1940), p. 259.
19. Hans Reichenback, *Atom and Cosmos: The World of Modern Physics* (New York: Macmillan, 1933), p. 270.
20. Barry Commoner, *The Closing Circle* (New York: Knopf, 1971), p. 189.
21. Peter Sedgwick, "Illness—Mental and Otherwise," *Hastings Center Studies*, vol. 1, no. 3 (1973), pp. 30, 31.
22. Chester R. Burns, "Disease Versus Healths: Some Legacies in the Philosophies of Modern Medical Science," in *Evaluation and Explanation in the Biomedical Sciences*, e. H. T. Englehardt and S. Spicker (Boston: D. Reidel Publishing Co., 1975), pp. 29ff.

23. Illich, pp. 15–17.
24. Leon Kass, "Regarding the End of Medicine and the Pursuit of Health," *The Public Interest*, no. 40, Summer 1975, p. 23.
25. Mark Zborowski, *People in Pain* (San Francisco: Jossey-Bass, 1969),p. 67.
26. Aarne Siirala, *The Voice of Illness* (Philadelphia: Fortress Press, 1969), pp. 58, 59.
27. Leo Tolstoy, "The Death of Ivan Illyich," in *Leo Tolstoy, Short Stories*, trans. Margaret Wettlin (Moscow: Progress Publishers, n.d.), pp. 108–167.
28. William Faulkner, "The Kingdom of God," New Orleans *Times-Picayune*, April 25, 1925.
29. Charles D. Peavy, "The Eyes of Innocence: Faulkner's 'The Kingdom of God'," *Papers on Language and Literature* (PLL), vol. 2, no. 2., Spring 1966, pp. 178–182.
30. Jerome Lejeune, "Discussion," in *Ethical Issues in Human Genetics*, ed. Bruce Hilton and Daniel Callahan (New York: Plenum, 1973), p. 113.
31. Barnabas Ahern, *New Horizons* (Notre Dame, Ind.: Fides Press, 1963).
32. Friedrich Schliermacher, *The Christian Faith* (Edinburgh: Black, 1948), p. 126.

IV. THE RENOVATION

1. From *Amahl and the Night Visitors* by Gian-Carlo Menotti. Copyright 1952 by Gian-Carlo Menotti. Used with permission of McGraw-HillBook Company.
2. Illich, p. 211.
3. Gregory Zilborg and George Henry, *History of Medical Psychology* (New York: Norton, 1941), p. 278.
4. See, for example, James Gustafson, *The Contributions of Theology to Medical Ethics* (Milwaukee, Wisc.: Marquette University Press, 1975).
5. René Dubos, *A God Within* (New York: Scribner's, 1972), p. 174.
6. Louis Pasteur, quoted in Garlick, p. 215.
7. Gunther Stent, "Molecular Biology and Metaphysics," *Nature*, vol. 248, April 26, 1974, p. 779. See also Edward O. Dodson, "Further Thoughts on Molecular Biology and Metaphysics," *Perspectives in Biology and Medicine*, vol. 18, no. 3, Spring 1974, pp. 306ff.
8. Buckminster Fuller, *Synergetics: Explorations in the Geometry of Thinking* (New York: Macmillan, 1975).
9. Pico della Mirandola, quoted in Ernst Cassirer, *The Renaissance Philosophy of Man* (Chicago: University of Chicago Press, 1948), pp. 224–225.
10. Kazoh Kitamori, *Theology of the Pain of God* (Richmond, Va.: John Knox Press, 1965), pp. 80ff.
11. Paul Tillich, *Systematische Theologie, V. II* (Stuttgart: Evangelisches Verlagswerk, 1958), p. 80. Author's translation.
12. Simone Weil, *Gravity and Grace* (New York: Putnam's, 1952), p. 197.

13. Dorothee Sölle, *Suffering* (Philadelphia: Fortress Press, 1975), p. 108.
14. "Optimum Care for Hopelessly Ill Patients: A Report of the Clinical Care Committee of the Massachusetts General Hospital," *New England Journal of Medicine,* vol. 295, no. 7, August 12, 1976, pp. 362ff.
15. Hippocrates quoted in the René Dubos, *Man, Medicine and Environment* (New York: Praeger, 1968), pp. 82, 83.
16. Thomas Mann, *The Magic Mountain* (New York: Knopf, 1951), p. 66. Somerset Maugham, "The Summing Up," in *The Maugham Reader* (Garden City, N.Y.: Doubleday, 1950), pp. 486–489.
18. Wolff, H. G., S. Wolf, and C. C. Hare, eds., *Life Stress and Bodily Disease* (Baltimore, Md.: Wilkens and Wilkens, 1950).
19. Thomas Holmes, "Life Crisis and Disease Onset: Qualifications and Quantitative Definition of the Life Crisis and Its Association With Health Change," privately distributed paper, 1974, p. 4. A concise review of the work of Holmes is found in T. Holmes and M. Masuda, "Life Change and Illness Susceptibility," in *Separation and Depression*, (New York: American Academy for the Advancement of Science, 1973), pp. 161–186.
20. Rollo May, *Love and Will* (New York: Dell, 1969), p. 21.
21. Otho T. Beall and Richard H. Shryock, *Cotton Mather: First Significant Figure in American Medicine* (Baltimore, Md.: Johns Hopkins Press, 1954).
22. Cotton Mather, quoted in *The American Heritage History of the Thirteen Colonies*, ed. M. Blow (New York: American Heritage, 1967), pp. 237, 238. Courtesy of the Massachusetts Historical Society.
23. Loren Eiseley, quoted in *U.S. News and World Report*, March 3, 1975, p. 43.
24. Jürgen Moltmann, "Hope and the Biomedical Future of Man," in *Hope and the Future of Man*, ed. Ewert Cousins (Philadelphia: Fortress Press, 1972), p. 104.
25. Sölle, p. 38.
26. Kitamori, p. 98.
27. George W. Kosmak, "The Training of Medical Students in Obstetrics," *Proceedings of the Annual Congress of Medical Education*, (1936), pp. 15–18.
28. Henri Nouwen, *The Wounded Healer* (Garden City, N.Y.: Doubleday, 1972).
29. Robert Jay Lifton, *History and Human Survival* (New York: Random House, 1970), p. 318.
30. Robert Jay Lifton, *Boundaries* (New York: Random House, 1970), p. 22.
31. Nouwen, p. 91.

Topical Bibliography

I. THEOLOGY AND MEDICINE

Altner, Gunter, ed. *The Human Creature*. Doubleday, Garden City, N.Y., 1974.

Becker, Ernest. *Revolution in Psychiatry: The New Understanding of Man*. Free Press, New York, 1974.

Boisen, Anton. *Exploration of the Inner World: A Study of Mental Disorder and Religious Experience*. Harper & Row, New York, 1936.

——. *Out of the Depths: An Autobiographical Study of Mental Disorder and Religious Experience*. Harper & Row, New York, 1960.

Brown, W. *Mind, Medicine and Metaphysics*. Oxford University Press, Oxford, 1936.

Browne, Thomas. *Religio Medici*. Cambridge University Press, Cambridge, England, 1963.

Bultmann, Rudolph, ed. *Life and Death*. A. C. Black, London, 1965.

Hiltner, Seward. *Religion and Health*. Macmillan, New York, 1943.

Kitamori, Kazoh. *Theology and the Pain of God*. John Knox Press, Richmond, Va., 1965.

May, William E. *Becoming Human: An Invitation to Christian Ethics*. Pflaum, Dayton, Ohio, 1975.

Raven, Charles. *Science, Medicine, and Morals*. Hodder and Stoughton, London, 1959.

Wise, Carrol. *Religion in Illness and Health*. Harper & Row, New York, 1942.

II. THEODICY/EVIL IN CREATION

Boras, Ladislaus. *Pain and Providence*. Helicon, Baltimore, Md., 1966.

Buttrick, G. A. *God, Pain and Evil*. Abingdon Press, Nashville, Tenn., 1966.

Ferre, Nels F. S. *Evil and the Christian Faith*. Harper & Row, New York, 1947.

Finch, William. *God and Evil*. Eerdmans, Grand Rapids, Mich., 1967.

Hartshorn, Charles. *Natural Theology For Our Time*. Open Court, New York, 1967.

Hick, J. *Evil and the God of Love*. Harper & Row, New York, 1966.

King, A. R. *The Problem of Evil*. Ronald Press, New York, 1952.

Lavelle, Louis. *Evil and Suffering*. Macmillan, New York, 1963.

III. SUFFERING

Beecher, Henry. "Relationship of Significance of Wound to the Pain Experience," *JAMA* 161: 1609–13, 1956.

Bowker, John. *The Problem of Suffering in the Religions of the World*. Cambridge University Press, Cambridge, England, 1970.

Fitch, Robert. *Of Love and Suffering*. Westminster, Philadelphia, 1971.

Kierkegaard, Soren. *The Gospel of Suffering and the Lilies of the Field*. Augsburg, Minneapolis, Minn., 1948.

Kübler-Ross, Elisabeth. *On Death and Dying*. Macmillan, New York, 1969.

Lewis, C. S. *The Problem of Pain*. Macmillan, New York, 1943.

McGill, A. *Suffering: A Test of Theological Method*. Geneva Press, Philadelphia, 1968.

Moltmann, Jürgen. *The Crucified God*. Harper & Row, New York, 1974.

Oates, W. E. *The Revelation of God in Human Suffering*. Westminster, Philadelphia, 1952.

Peake, A. S. *The Problem of Suffering in the Old Testament*. Epworth Press, London, 1947.

Stringfellow, W. *A Second Birthday*. Doubleday, Garden City, N.Y., 1970.

Taylor, Michael J. *The Mystery of Suffering and Death*. Alba House, New York, 1973.

Thielicke, Helmut. *Death and Life*. Fortress Press, Philadelphia, 1970.

Zborowski, Mark. *People in Pain*. Jossey-Bass, San Francisco, 1969.

IV. SIN AND SICKNESS

Bakan, David. *Disease, Pain and Sacrifice*. Beacon, Boston, 1971.

Haring, Bernard. *Sin in the Secular Age*. Doubleday, Garden City, N.Y., 1974.

Rather, Lelland J. *Disease, Life and Man*. Stanford University Press, Stanford, Calif., 1958.

von Weizsacker, Victor. *Der Kranke Mensch*. Kaiser Verlag, Stuttgart, 1951.

V. THE NATURE OF HEALTH

Dicks, Russell Leslie. *Thy Health Shall Spring Forth*. Macmillan, New York, 1945.

Dubos, René. *Beast or Angel: Choices That Make Us Human*. Scribner's, New York, 1974.

———and Pynes, Maya. *Health and Disease*. Time-Life Books, New York, 1965.

Lapsley, James. *Salvation and Health: The Interlocking Processes of Life*. Westminster, Philadelphia, 1972.

Pieper, Josef. *Happiness and Contemplation*. Pantheon, New York, 1958.

Russell, Leslie. *Toward Health and Wholeness*. Macmillan, New York, 1964.

Sinacore, John S. *Health, A Quality of Life*. Macmillan, New York, 1968.

VI. HEALING

Ackerknecht, Erwin H. *Therapeutics: From the Primitives to the Twentieth Century*. Hafner Press, New York, 1973.

Dawson, George. *Healing, Pagan and Christian*. Macmillan, New York, 1935.

Doniger, Simon, ed. *Healing: Human and Divine*. Association Press, New York, 1957.

Frazier, Claude, ed. *Faith Healing, Finger of God or Scientific Curiosity*. Nelson, New York, 1973.

———. *Healing and Religious Faith*. United Church Press, Philadelphia, 1974.

Frost, Evelyn. *Christian Healing*. A. R. Mowbray, London, 1940.

Goldbrinner, Josef. *Holiness Is Wholeness*. Notre Dame Press, South Bend, Ind., 1964.

126   TOPICAL BIBLIOGRAPHY

Hempel, Johannes. *Heilung als Symbol und Wirklichkeit im biblischen Schrifttum*. Vandenhoeck und Ruprecht, Göttigen, 1958.
Hoch, Dorothee. *Healing and Salvation*. SCM Press, London, 1958.
Kelsey, Morton T. *Healing and Christianity*. Harper & Row, New York, 1973.
Kiev, Ari, ed. *Magic, Faith and Healing*. Free Press, New York, 1964.
Lynch, William. *Images of Hope*. Notre Dame Press, South Bend, Ind., 1974.
Naegele, Kaspar D. *Health and Healing*. Jossey-Bass, San Francisco, 1970.
Nouwen, Henri. *The Wounded Healer: Ministry in a Contemporary Society*. Doubleday, Garden City, N.Y., 1972.
Peterman, Mary E. *Healing and Spiritual Adventure*. Fortress Press, Philadelphia, 1974.
Scharlemann, Marton Henry. *Healing and Redemption*. Concordia Publishing House, St. Louis, Mo., 1965.

VII. MENTAL HEALTH

Foucault, Michel. *Madness and Civilization*. Pantheon, New York, 1965.
Frankl, Victor. *The Doctor and the Soul*. Knopf, New York, 1939.
Goldbrinner, Josef. *Cure of Mind and Cure of Soul*. Pantheon, New York, 1958.
Hoffman, Hans. *Religion and Mental Health*. Harper & Row, New York, 1961.
Kenny, Anthony. *The Anatomy of the Soul: Historical Essays in the Philosophy of Mind*. Western Printing Services, Bristol, England, 1973.
May, Rollo. *Man's Search for Himself*. Norton, New York, 1953.

VIII. HISTORY OF INTERPRETATION OF HEALTH AND DISEASE

Ayala, Francisco Jose and Dobzhansky, Theodosious, ed. *Studies in the Philosophy of Biology Reduction and Related Problems*. University of California Press, Berkeley, Calif., 1974.
Camp, John. *Magic, Myth and Medicine*. Gaplinger, New York, 1974.
Dubos, René. *Man, Medicine and Environment*. Praeger, New York, 1968.

Garlick, Phillis. *Man's Search for Health*. The Highway Press, London, 1952.

Herzlich, Claudine. *Health and Illness: Social Psychological Analysis*. Academe Press, London, 1973.

Illich, Ivan. *Medical Nemesis*. Pantheon, New York, 1976.

Jayne, Walter Addison. *The Healing Gods of Ancient Civilizations*. New York University Books, New Hyde Park, N.Y., 1962.

McCasland, S. Vernon. *By the Finger of God: Demon Possession and Exorcism in Early Christianity*. Macmillan, New York, 1951.

McNeill, John T. *A History of the Cure of Souls*. Harper & Row, New York, 1951.

Riese, Walter. *The Conception of Disease: Its History, Its Versions and Its Nature*. Philosophical Library, New York, 1953.

Trilling, Lionel. *Freud and the Crisis of Our Culture*. Beacon, Boston, 1955.

Zilboorg, Gregory. *The Medical Man and the Witch During the Renaissance*. Johns Hopkins Press, Baltimore, Md., 1935.

Index